Quick & Easy
400-CALORIE RECIPES

Quarto.com

© 2024 Quarto Publishing Group USA Inc.
Text © 2011 Dick Logue

First Published in 2024 by New Shoe Press, an imprint of The Quarto Group,
100 Cummings Center, Suite 265-D, Beverly, MA 01915, USA.
T (978) 282-9590 F (978) 283-2742

Essential, In-Demand Topics, Four-Color Design, Affordable Price
New Shoe Press publishes affordable, beautifully designed books covering evergreen, in-demand subjects. With a goal to inform and inspire readers' everyday hobbies, from cooking and gardening to wellness and health to art and crafts, New Shoe titles offer the ultimate library of purposeful, how-to guidance aimed at meeting the unique needs of each reader. Reimagined and redesigned from Quarto's best-selling backlist, New Shoe books provide practical knowledge and opportunities for all DIY enthusiasts to enrich and enjoy their lives.

Visit Quarto.com/New-Shoe-Press for a complete listing of the New Shoe Press books.

New Shoe Press titles are also available at discount for retail, wholesale, promotional, and bulk purchase. For details, contact the Special Sales Manager by email at specialsales@quarto.com or by mail at The Quarto Group, Attn: Special Sales Manager, 100 Cummings Center, Suite 265-D, Beverly, MA 01915, USA.

10 9 8 7 6 5 4 3 2 1

ISBN: 978-0-7603-9052-8
eISBN: 978-0-7603-9053-5

The content in this book was previously published in *500 400-Calorie Recipes* (2011 Fair Winds Press) by Dick Logue.

Library of Congress Cataloging-in-Publication Data available

Printed in China

The information in this book is for educational purposes only. It is not intended to replace the advice of a physician or medical practitioner. Please see your health-care provider before beginning any new health program.

Quick & Easy
400-CALORIE RECIPES

Delicious and Satisfying Meals That Keep You to a Balanced 1200-Calorie Diet So You Can Lose Weight Without Starving Yourself

DICK LOGUE

NEW SHOE PRESS

Contents

Introduction

Why 400-Calorie Recipes?

No doubt that is the first question that came to your mind when you saw this book. The answer is simple, a 400-calorie meal is just what you need to lose weight, a meal that satisfies you and keeps your hunger at bay until the next meal but only contains 400 calories. You might call them "mega." Of course, there is more to it than that. The goal of our meals is to help you be healthier, lose weight, and do it all without feeling deprived or hungry.

Does this sound too good to be true? It's not! The key is to eat foods that contain all the nutrients you need and that stick with you until the next meal. Each meal we offer here is approximately 400 calories, so you can eat three of these filling meals, or even four, and still only get 1200 to 1600 calories per day. In the next chapter, we'll explore in detail how all this works, talking about calories, nutrient density, and the kind of foods you should and should not be eating. But for now all you need to know is that it does work.

This is not something that I created. It is based on the research of a number of doctors and nutritional experts. One of the most important is Dr. Barbara Rolls, a professor of nutrition at the University of Pennsylvania. Dr. Rolls has published a number of articles and research papers on the subject of diet and weight loss. She says that people feel full because of the amount of food they eat not because of the number of calories or the grams of fat, protein, or carbohydrates. So the trick is to fill up on foods that aren't full of calories. She has done a number of experiments to confirm her findings. She found that given free choice, people tended to eat the same *amount* of food each day. By varying the amount of high volume, low calorie foods compared to high calorie, low volume foods, people were able to eat the same amount and feel just as satisfied while eating

as much as 400 fewer calories per day. She uses the term *energy density* to describe the number of calories in a given quantity of food.

In order to see how significant this is, let's take a quick look at how people lose weight. There are lots of different diets and lots of different theories, but the bottom line is that if we burn more calories than we take in, we lose weight. If we eat more calories than our bodies use, we gain weight. About 3500 calories is equivalent to a pound. So in order to lose a pound a week, we need to keep our calorie intake to about 500 calories a day less than our bodies use. So Dr. Rolls' findings mean that people could lose almost a pound a week not even watching how *much* they eat, just replacing some of the foods with high energy density with other foods with lower energy density. An example is a pasta salad. If it contains a lot of pasta compared to vegetables, it will have a high energy density. If you replace some of the pasta with additional vegetables you will still have the same volume of food and feel just as satisfied but with fewer calories. That is one of the main concepts that went into creating these recipes.

So the obvious question is how many calories we burn in a day. There isn't any simple answer. It depends on a number of factors including age, gender, activity level, and your current weight and height. There are a number of sites online that contain a calorie needs calculator that will do your specific calculation. But I can tell you this, no matter what I put into them I didn't come up with anything less than 1500 calories per day. That figure was for a small, older, sedentary woman. For my own calculation, I came up with more than 2200 per day to maintain my weight.

So how does all that relate to this book? I'm suggesting that if you want to lose weight, you can eat three satisfying meals a day of about 400 calories each, maybe throw in a healthy snack or two, and end up with a total daily calorie count of less than 1500 calories. In my case, that would translate to a weight loss of about a pound and a half (0.68 kg) a week. Of course as the auto commercials used to say "your mileage may vary". Your answers to the calorie calculator are going to be different than mine and your expected weight loss will be different. But unless you are a person already so thin that you don't need to lose weight, you will almost certainly be eating fewer calories than you burn.

Of course it isn't quite that simple. Since I came to create recipes because of a need to eat heart healthy food, I have some ideas about how we should structure these mega meals for maximum health, not just weight loss. In the next section, we'll discuss some of those.

Our Approach to Weight Loss

I've identified six key areas that I looked at as I created these recipes. As I said, the goal is a healthy diet that will help you to lose weight. We'll look at each of those areas in more detail in the next chapter.

Low Energy Density

We can eat the healthiest diet imaginable, but if we eat too many calories we aren't going to lose weight. That statement isn't quite true. The other concepts of healthy eating actually support this goal also.

High fat foods are generally unhealthy to eat. They also provide more calories for a given quantity of food. Fiber contains few calories, so high fiber foods are not only good for you, but they are also a way to speed your weight loss.

High Nutrient Density

This is in some ways the opposite of energy density. What it measures is the amount of nutrients in a specific quantity of a given food. A system of rating nutrient density called the Aggregate Nutrient Density Index (ANDI) was developed by Dr. Joel Fuhrman, a New Jersey physician who specializes in preventing and reversing disease through nutrition. The rankings are based not only on vitamins and minerals but also phytochemicals, compounds that are thought to promote good health but have not been established as essential nutrients. This includes things that you have probably heard of like antioxidants and beta carotene.

Focus on Fresh, Minimally Processed Foods

There has been an increased focus on avoiding processed foods in recent years. This has resulted in things like the caveman diet and Paleolithic diets. I'm not going to go so far as to suggest that, but I will say that I believe processing reduces natural nutrients and replaces them with chemicals, some of questionable safety. The Canyon Ranch spa cookbook I own suggests "Don't eat anything your great-grandmother didn't," and that seems like a reasonable approach to me. That being said, I do use artificial sweeteners to help hold down the calories in some recipes with significant amounts of sugar, so I do make compromises.

Low Sodium

Some of you may know (especially if you've skipped ahead to the next section) that I got started creating recipes and eventually writing books because I was on a low sodium diet for congestive heart failure and I was dissatisfied with the kind of food I could eat. Not all of the recipes here are as strictly low in sodium as my personal diet. I've used regular baking powder and cheese and included a few recipes with ham and other high sodium ingredients. But I'm still convinced that most people get more sodium in their diet than they really need.

Low Saturated Fat

To a large degree I've tried to hold down the total fat level in these recipes as much as is practical. But all fat is not created equal. Fats such as those found in olive and canola oil and vegetables like avocados may actually be beneficial. But it is pretty much universally accepted that both saturated and trans fats represent health risks and I have tried to limit them as much as possible.

High Fiber

Eating foods high in fiber is another of those things that has multiple positive effects. In the first place, it's healthy from both the heart and digestive point of view. But it also plays a part in our attempts to lower the energy density of meals. Fiber-rich foods such as legumes and whole grains tend to have a lower energy density and a higher nutrient density, so that's good all around.

How This Book Came About

Some of you may already know about me, either from my website or from the other books I've written. If so, you know that I have focused primarily on heart healthy cooking. I started thinking about low sodium cooking after being diagnosed with congestive heart failure in 1999. One of the first and biggest things I had to deal with was the doctor's insistence that I follow a low sodium

diet . . . 1200 mg a day or less. At first, like many people, I found it easiest to just avoid the things that had a lot of sodium in them. But I was bored. And I was convinced that there had to be a way to create low sodium versions of the food I missed. So I learned all kinds of new ways to cook things. I researched where to get low sodium substitutes for the things that I couldn't have any more, bought cookbooks, and basically redid my whole diet.

Along the way, I learned some things. And I decided to try to share this information with others who were in the same position I had been in. I started a website, www.lowsodiumcooking.com, to share recipes and information. I sent out an email newsletter with recipes that now has over 20,000 subscribers. And I wrote my first book, *500 Low Sodium Recipes*.

By that time I had progressed to other areas of interest in healthy cooking. When my cholesterol became too high to please my cardiologist, I had to learn about low cholesterol cooking. When I was told that my blood sugar levels indicated that I was a borderline diabetic, I became interested in the role of carbohydrates in your diet. I became more aware of the work that had been done on glycemic index and glycemic load and began incorporating these concepts into the food we prepared and ate. Both of these interests turned into another 500 recipes book.

But I was also concerned about my weight. And so was my wife. I was following the exercise plan my doctor had given me, but I wasn't able to lose those last 10 pounds or so that I wanted to, even though I thought I was cooking healthy meals. So once more, I went back to the research. And there I discovered the work of Dr. Rolls and others with similar ideas. So we began incorporating these concepts into our cooking. It turns out it was easy to maintain a heart healthy diet while looking at nutrient density. Many of the same things that made food heart healthy also made it a good choice for these meals. And as we began to pay more attention to these ideas and began to lose that weight that had been so stubborn, the idea of another book developed. And here it is, 500 mega meals to get you started on losing weight and feeling better.

How Is the Nutritional Information Calculated?

The nutritional information included with these recipes was calculated using the AccuChef program. It calculates the values using the latest U.S. Department of Agriculture Standard reference nutritional database. I've been using this program since I first started trying to figure out how much sodium was in the recipes I've created. It's inexpensive, easy to use, and has a number of really handy features. For instance, if I go in and change the nutrition figures for an ingredient, it remembers those figures whenever I use that ingredient. AccuChef is available online from www.accuchef.com. They offer a free trial version if you want to try it out, and the full version costs less than $20US.

Of course, that implies that these figures are estimates. Every brand of tomatoes or any other product is a little different in nutritional content. These figures were calculated using products that I buy in southern Maryland. If you use a different brand, your nutrition figures may be different. Use the nutritional analysis as a guideline in determining whether a recipe is right for your diet.

Where's the Salt?

One question that may occur to some people looking over the recipes in this book is "Why is there no salt in any of the ingredient lists?" That's a fair question and deserves an answer. As I said in the Introduction, I first got involved with healthy cooking because my doctor put me on a low sodium diet. It took some time and lots of experimentation, but I learned how to cook things that both taste good and are easy to prepare that are still low in sodium. Along the way we literally threw away our saltshaker. There's one shaker of light salt, which is half salt and half salt substitute, on the table. My wife uses that occasionally. Two of my children have given up salt completely, not because they need to for medical reasons, but because they are convinced like I am that it's the healthy thing to do. When I started looking at creating 400-calorie meal recipes, going back to using salt wasn't even something I considered.

Most Americans get far more than the 2300 mg of sodium a day recommended for a healthy adult. This happens without our even thinking about it. In creating these recipes, I was not as strict about the amount of sodium as I usually am. But I also didn't add any salt. I think if you try the recipes you'll find that they taste good without it. If you are tempted to add some salt because you think it's needed, I'd suggest you check with your doctor first. I believe that most of them will agree that in the interest of total health, you are better off without the salt.

Changing the Way You Think about What You Eat

To a large degree, this book is a starting point. Here we are going to look at each of the six areas we talked about in the introduction in more detail.

Energy Density

Let's look in a little more detail at the idea of energy density that we introduced previously. Energy density is defined as the number of calories in a gram of food. Dr. Rolls introduces a simple way to estimate that for items containing a nutrition label. The label contains both the number of calories and the number of grams in a serving, making a comparison relatively easy. If the number of calories is less than the number of grams in a serving, that food in general has a low energy density and can be eaten freely. This category includes many fruits and vegetables, nonfat dairy products, and soups. If the number of calories is between 1 and 2 times the number of grams, you should be aware of the amount you eat and be strict about portion control. This group includes starchy vegetables, low fat meats, and many bean and grain products. The closer the ratio is to 2, the more careful you should be. If the number of calories is more than twice the number of grams, you should limit how much you eat. This includes fried foods, butter and oil, and candies.

Another way to look at this is in terms of the basic food building blocks and how many calories they contain. At the top end are fats, which contain 9 calories per gram. We obviously want to limit those. Carbohydrates contain about 4 calories per gram, less than half that of fat. Fiber contains only 2 calories per gram. Water contains none at all. This is why many of the recipes in this book contain lots of vegetables that contain a high percentage of water like zucchini and eggplant. This is free volume for your diet; it helps to fill you up without providing any calories.

Nutrient Density

Nutrient density was a key element in creating these recipes. If we are going to reduce the number of calories we take in, we want to make sure that we still get all the nutrition we need. In many cases, the same foods that have low energy density have high nutrient density, so that is a help. In looking at nutrient density, one of the things I looked at was the information that was published by Dr. Fuhrman. His ANDI scale calculates nutrient density based on a number of vitamins, minerals, and other nutrients in food, coming up with a way of comparing different foods to see which have the most nutrients for a specific quantity. His general recommendation is to focus on bright colored plant products. Green leafy vegetables rate near the top of the list, as do things like carrots, tomatoes, and strawberries. The bottom of the list contains things like oils, processed grain products like bread and pasta, dairy products, and meats.

Focus on Fresh Foods

What we have to say here mirrors much of the other things we've said in this chapter. The idea is that processing takes away the nutrient content of food. So the best thing you can do for both the nutrient density of food and the freshness is to process it as little as possible. A couple of quick guidelines:

Sodium

To me this is obvious and second nature. After 11 years on a low sodium diet I can't imagine eating any other way. The fact that I feel so much better now than I did when I first started it is enough proof for me. I've tried not to be a fanatic about sodium content in these recipes. There are a couple that have almost as much sodium as I'm allowed daily. I don't eat those. But I'm not going to tell you that you shouldn't. But as I said in the Where's the Salt section in the introduction, I don't add salt to things. Ever. So if you feel the need to, you'll have to do that on your own.

Fats

Another of those areas that are good news for multiple reasons is the reduction of fats. There are two main types of fats we want to limit: saturated fat and trans fats. In general, saturated fats are fats that are solid at room temperature. There are several categories of saturated fats. In each case, there are better alternatives or things we can do to reduce the fat. The recipes in this book are designed with that in mind.

Trans fats are also called trans-fatty acids. They are produced by adding hydrogen to vegetable oil through a process called hydrogenation. This makes the fat more solid and less likely to spoil. Although increased awareness of their health risks have started to reduce their use, trans fat are still a common ingredient in commercial baked goods and fried foods. Food manufacturers are required to list trans fat content on nutrition labels.

Fiber

As we already saw, foods that are high in fiber are generally lower in energy density, so that a good thing for us right out of the gate. But there are some other health benefits of increasing the fiber in your diet.

Things We Want More of In Our Healthy Diet

Based on the above can list, a couple of general guidelines for things that we want to see more of in our diet:
- Whole foods such as produce and fresh meats
- Brightly colored fruits and vegetables
- Whole grains
- Legumes, including lentils, soybeans, dried peas, and beans

Things We Want Less of

We can also come up with a high level list of those things that we want to limit:
- Refined, processed foods such as white flour and sugar
- Packaged foods, which often contain ingredients you would be better off without
- Saturated fats and trans fats
- Empty calories, such as sweetened beverages and alcohol

And now on to the recipes!

Traditional Breakfasts

Are you a big breakfast fan (like me!)? And are you thinking that breakfast is going to be changed completely as you follow our new meal plan? Think again. Breakfast is just as important as any other meal in our new way of eating. In fact, it may be more important because it's the meal that gets you started on your path of feeling satisfied on fewer calories each day. And there are lots of recipes that contain eggs and other traditional breakfast foods but still adhere to our principles.

Fill Yourself Up but Not Out Breakfast Casserole

This is a fairly traditional breakfast casserole. Well, except for the chilies, which do add a little flavor and heat. Along with those, it contains a generous helping of other vegetables to keep you going through the morning.

24 ounces (680 g) frozen hash browns

1 cup (233 ml) skim milk

1 cup (235 ml) egg substitute

½ cup (80 g) onion, diced

½ cup (75 g) red bell pepper

4 ounces (115 g) diced green chilies

¾ cup (83 g) Swiss cheese, grated

6 slices low sodium bacon, cooked and crumbled

Spray a 9 × 13 inch (23 × 33 cm) pan with nonstick vegetable oil spray. Add hash browns. Cook in 350°F (180°C, or gas mark 4) oven for 20 minutes. Mix all remaining ingredients, pour over potatoes, and cook for 30 more minutes.

—

6 servings

Each with: 414 Calories (48% from Fat, 17% from Protein, 35% from Carb); 18 g Protein; 23 g Total Fat; 9 g Saturated Fat; 9 g Monounsaturated Fat; 3 g Polyunsaturated Fat; 37 g Carb; 3 g Fiber; 3 g Sugar; 322 mg Phosphorus; 234 mg Calcium; 3 mg Iron; 230 mg Sodium; 811 mg Potassium; 763 IU Vitamin A; 61 mg ATE Vitamin E; 24 mg Vitamin C; 25 mg Cholesterol

Ham and Egg Casserole

This is a fairly typical ham and egg bake, except for the addition of the zucchini and mushrooms. They take the place of the more typical potatoes, which have significantly more calories.

2 tablespoons (28 g) unsalted butter, melted

1 pound (455 g) low fat Monterey Jack cheese, shredded

2½ cups (570 ml) egg substitute, beaten

2 tablespoons (16 g) all purpose flour

16 ounces (455 g) fat-free cottage cheese

2 cups (300 g) ham, cubed

⅛ teaspoon Tabasco sauce

1 teaspoon baking powder

1 cup (120 g) zucchini, shredded

8 ounces (225 g) mushrooms, sliced

1 cup (150 g) red bell pepper, chopped

Preheat oven to 400°F (200°C, or gas mark 6). Put butter in 9-inch (23 cm) pan and melt in oven. Combine all other ingredients and put in pan. Bake at 400°F (200°C, or gas mark 6) for 15 minutes and then at 350°F (180°C, or gas mark 4) degrees for 15 to 20 minutes more.

—

6 servings

Each with: 413 Calories (39% from Fat, 51% from Protein, 10% from Carb); 52 g Protein; 18 g Total Fat; 8 g Unsaturated Fat; 6 g Monounsaturated Fat; 3 g Polyunsaturated Fat; 10 g Carb; 1 g Fiber; 5 g Sugar; 764 mg Phosphorus; 471 mg Calcium; 1540 mg Sodium; 853 mg Potassium; 1503 IU Vitamin A; 85 mg ATE Vitamin E; 52 mg Vitamin C; 49 mg Cholesterol

Asparagus Omelet and Citrus Salad

This breakfast exemplifies what mega meals are all about. You get a large quantity of great tasting food without going over your calorie goals.

OMELET

10 ounces (280 g) asparagus, cut into ⅓-inch (8 mm) pieces

1½ cups (355 ml) egg substitute

⅓ cup (33 g) Parmesan cheese, finely grated

¼ teaspoon black pepper

¼ cup (25 g) scallion, thinly sliced

SALAD

6 ounces (170 g) mandarin oranges

2 grapefruits, cut into sections

3 cups (165 g) Bibb lettuce

6 tablespoons (90 g) poppy seed dressing

Steam the asparagus until crisp/tender, about 5 minutes, and drain. Whisk the egg substitute, grated Parmesan cheese, and black pepper in a large bowl to blend well. Spray a skillet with nonstick vegetable oil spray. Sauté sliced scallions for 3 minutes or until softened. Add cooked asparagus and sauté until heated through. Reduce heat to medium; spread the asparagus mixture in a single layer in the skillet. Pour the egg mixture over the asparagus. Cook until the eggs are softly set, tilting skillet and gently running a rubber spatula around the edge to allow uncooked egg to flow underneath, about 4 minutes. Slide the omelet out onto a plate, folding in half. Cut omelet into wedges and serve. While the omelet is cooking, combine mandarin oranges, grapefruit sections, and lettuce in a large salad bowl; toss lightly with dressing and divide onto salad plates.

—

3 servings

Each with: 388 Calories (43% from Fat, 24% from Protein, 32% from Carb); 24 g Protein; 19 g Total Fat; 4 g Saturated Fat; 2 g Monounsaturated Fat; 2 g Polyunsaturated Fat; 32 g Carb; 6 g Fiber; 25 g Sugar; 331 mg Phosphorus; 272 mg Calcium; 6 mg Iron; 906 mg Sodium; 1167 mg Potassium; 5667 IU Vitamin A; 13 mg ATE Vitamin E; 105 mg Vitamin C; 11 mg Cholesterol

Ready to Ride the Range Breakfast

This is a fairly spicy Southwestern breakfast that's full of flavor but within the limits of your diet. So enjoy yourself before saddling up and going off to work.

1 large potato

¾ pound (340 g) turkey sausage

1 small onion, chopped

1 teaspoon chili powder

¼ teaspoon cayenne pepper

¾ cup (175 ml) egg substitute

6 whole wheat tortillas, 8-inch (20 cm)

½ cup (58 g) reduced fat Monterey Jack cheese

½ cup (130 g) salsa

Cook the potato in boiling water 35 minutes until tender. (I cooked mine in the microwave.) When cool, peel and cut into cubes. Brown sausage in frying pan. Add chopped onion, chili powder, and cayenne pepper. Cook for 10 minutes. Drain and discard any fat. Add cubed, cooked potato. Beat egg substitute and add to pan. Stir until eggs are set. Spoon mixture into center of warmed tortilla, top with shredded cheese, and roll up tortilla to enclose mixture. Serve topped with salsa.

—
6 servings

Each with: 409 Calories (40% from Fat, 21% from Protein, 39% from Carb); 21 g Protein; 18 g Total Fat; 7 g Saturated Fat; 6 g Monounsaturated Fat; 3 g Polyunsaturated Fat; 40 g Carb; 3 g Fiber; 3 g Sugar; 297 mg Phosphorus; 191 mg Calcium; 767 mg Sodium; 640 mg Potassium; 502 IU Vitamin A; 21 mg ATE Vitamin E; 28 mg Vitamin C; 44 mg Cholesterol

Breakfast Enchiladas for Family and Guests

A make-ahead breakfast, you can assemble this the night before and then just bake it in the morning. This and the large number of servings make it a great choice when you have company staying overnight. Or just freeze the extras so you'll have it ready the next time you want it.

12 ounces (340 g) ham, finely chopped

½ cup (50 g) green onion, chopped

2 cups (300 g) green bell pepper, chopped

1 cup (160 g) onion, chopped

1½ cups (180 g) low fat cheddar cheese, grated

8 whole wheat tortillas, 8-inch (20 cm)

1½ cups (355 ml) egg substitute

2 cups (475 g) skim milk

1 tablespoon (8 g) all purpose flour

¼ teaspoon garlic powder

1 teaspoon Tabasco sauce

1 avocado

Preheat oven to 350°F (180°C, or gas mark 4). Mix together ham, onion, green bell pepper, and cheese. Divide mixture among tortillas and roll up. Place seam side down in a greased 12 × 7 × 2-inch (30 × 18 × 5 cm) pan. In separate bowl, beat egg substitute, skim milk, flour, garlic, and Tabasco sauce. Pour over enchiladas. Place in refrigerator overnight if desired. Cover with foil and bake for 30 minutes. Uncover for last 10 minutes. Top with slices of avocado to serve.

—
8 servings

Each with: 385 Calories (32% from Fat, 29% from Protein, 38% from Carb); 28 g Protein; 14 g Total Fat; 4 g Saturated Fat; 7 g Monounsaturated Fat; 2 g Polyunsaturated Fat; 37 g Carb; 4 g Fiber; 3 g Sugar; 425 mg Phosphorus; 291 mg Calcium; 951 mg Sodium; 716 mg Potassium; 587 IU Vitamin A; 52 mg ATE Vitamin E; 35 mg Vitamin C; 24 mg Cholesterol

Easy, Tasty, Filling Breakfast Strata

The title says it all. What more could you want? This is a great fix-head breakfast. We usually have some variation of this on holidays when there is a lot to do in the morning, but we want a special family breakfast.

1 pound (455 g) turkey sausage

2 cups (475 ml) egg substitute

10 slices whole wheat bread, cubed

3 cups (700 ml) skim milk

1 cup (115 g) low fat cheddar cheese, shredded

1 cup (160) onion, chopped

1 cup (150 g) red bell pepper, chopped

10 ounces (280 g) frozen chopped broccoli, thawed

2 tablespoons (28 g) unsalted butter, melted

2 tablespoons (16 g) all purpose flour

1 tablespoon (9 g) dry mustard

2 teaspoons dried basil

In large skillet, brown sausage. Drain. In large bowl, beat egg substitute. Add remaining ingredients and mix well. Spoon into greased 13 × 9-inch (33 × 23 cm) baking pan. Cover and refrigerate 8 hours or overnight. Preheat oven to 350°F (180°C, or gas mark 4). Bake 60 to 70 minutes or until knife inserted near center comes out clean.

—
8 servings

Each with: 391 Calories (42% from Fat, 29% from Protein, 29% from Carb); 29 g Protein; 18 g Total Fat; 7 g Saturated Fat; 5 g Monounsaturated Fat; 3 g Polyunsaturated Fat; 28 g Carb; 3 g Fiber; 4 g Sugar; 442 mg Phosphorus; 308 mg Calcium; 857 mg Sodium; 691 mg Potassium; 1534 IU Vitamin A; 90 mg ATE Vitamin E; 69 mg Vitamin C; 48 mg Cholesterol

Breakfast Quesadilla

This is a fairly traditional breakfast quesadilla, but it has the increased nutrition of added vegetables.

1 slice low sodium bacon

¼ cup (40 g) onion, chopped

½ cup (75 g) red bell pepper, chopped

¼ cup (60 ml) egg substitute

2 tablespoons (22 g) black beans

1 ounce (28 g) fat-free sour cream, divided

3 tablespoons (49 g) salsa, divided

1 whole wheat tortilla, 6-inch (15 cm)

¾ ounce (21 g) Swiss cheese

—
1 serving

Each with: 400 Calories (34% from Fat, 22% from Protein, 44% from Carb); 22 g Protein; 15 g Total Fat; 7 g Unsaturated Fat; 5 g Monounsaturated Fat; 2 g Polyunsaturated Fat; 45 g Carb; 6 g Fiber; 9 g Sugar; 380 mg Phosphorus; 362 mg Calcium; 786 mg Sodium; 788 mg Potassium; 3168 IU Vitamin A; 73 mg ATE Vitamin E; 152 mg Vitamin C; 31 mg Cholesterol

Cook bacon according to package directions, either in a pan with nonstick vegetable oil spray or in the microwave. Once cool enough to handle, roughly chop and set aside. Bring a medium large pan (at least the size of the tortilla) sprayed with nonstick vegetable oil spray to medium heat. Add the red bell pepper and onion and cook until softened, about 3 minutes. Add egg substitute and scramble until fully cooked. Transfer mixture to a bowl and set pan aside to cool. Add bacon, beans, 1 tablespoon (15 g) sour cream and 1 tablespoon (16 g) salsa to the egg scramble bowl. Lightly mix and set aside. Clean and dry the pan, spray with nonstick vegetable oil spray, and bring to medium-high heat. Place tortilla flat in the pan and sprinkle evenly with cheese. Spoon egg mixture over one half of the tortilla, fold the other half over the mixture to form the quesadilla, and then press down with a spatula to seal. Cook until both sides are crispy, about 2 minutes per side. Top with remaining salsa and sour cream.

Cheese and Vegetable Frittata

This is one of those recipes that ended up being quite a bit fewer than 400 calories. But if we put any more vegetables in it, it wouldn't fit in the pan. As low as it is, I guarantee you won't go away hungry.

2 cups (200 g) fresh green beans

1 cup (130) carrot, chopped

1 cup (100 g) cauliflower florets

¼ cup (80 g) onion, chopped

8 ounces (225 g) spinach

½ cup (75 g) green bell pepper, diced

½ cup (120 ml) egg substitute

1 cup (235 ml) fat-free evaporated milk

¼ cup (60 ml) water

1¾ cups (205 g) low fat cheddar cheese, shredded

⅛ teaspoon black pepper

Steam the vegetables for about 5 minutes, just to soften a little. In a mixing bowl, beat the egg substitute with the evaporated milk and water. Add ¾ cup (90 g) cheese and black pepper and mix well. Place the vegetables in an 8 × 8-inch (20 × 20 cm) glass baking dish. Cool slightly and then pour the liquid over. Sprinkle with remaining cheese. Bake for about 35 minutes at 375°F (190°C, or gas mark 5).

—
4 servings

Each with: 234 Calories (22% from Fat, 44% from Protein, 35% from Carb); 26 g Protein; 6 g Total Fat; 3 g Unsaturated Fat; 2 g Monounsaturated Fat; 1 g Polyunsaturated Fat; 21 g Carb; 5 g Fiber; 12 g Sugar; 519 mg Phosphorus; 538 mg Calcium; 559 mg Sodium; 979 mg Potassium; 10 108 IU Vitamin A; 110 mg ATE Vitamin E; 57 mg Vitamin C; 15 mg Cholesterol

Tortillas for Breakfast

And why not have tortillas for breakfast? These are made in a style like enchiladas. Extra lean ground beef adds a flavor boost while allowing the calories to stay low. Lots of veggies and eggs provide the bulk and the nutrition.

2 teaspoons olive oil

1 cup (160 g) onion, chopped

¾ pound (340 g) extra lean ground beef

1 cup (150 g) green bell pepper, chopped

¼ teaspoon black pepper

1½ cups (355 ml) egg substitute

6 whole wheat tortillas, 8-inch (20 cm)

½ cup (115 g) fat-free sour cream

½ cup (130 g) salsa

Heat oil in large fry pan. Add chopped onion, beef, green bell pepper, and black pepper. Stir-fry until tender. Pour egg substitute over onion mix and cook until half-cooked. Spoon into tortilla shells and roll. Bake at 350°F (180°C, or gas mark 4) for 25 minutes. Top with sour cream and salsa and bake 5 to 10 minutes longer.

—
6 servings

Each with: 397 Calories (44% from Fat, 24% from Protein, 32% from Carb); 23 g Protein; 19 g Total Fat; 7 g Unsaturated Fat; 8 g Monounsaturated Fat; 2 g Polyunsaturated Fat; 32 g Carb; 3 g Fiber; 3 g Sugar; 250 mg Phosphorus; 130 mg Calcium; 470 mg Sodium; 583 mg Potassium; 538 IU Vitamin A; 20 mg ATE Vitamin E; 25 mg Vitamin C; 48 mg Cholesterol

Chile Relleno Casserole

Chili relleno is not a dish that we usually associate with breakfast, but adding extra egg turns it into a breakfast full of flavor and nutrition.

4 ounces (115 g) green chili peppers, whole

8 ounces (225 g) low fat cheddar cheese, grated

4 ounces (115 g) low fat Monterey Jack cheese, grated

1 cup (235 ml) egg substitute

2 tablespoons (16 g) all purpose flour

14 ounces (425 ml) fat-free evaporated milk

Rinse chilies and remove seeds. Place half the chilies in a greased casserole dish. Sprinkle half of both cheeses on top and add remaining chilies. Top with remaining cheese. Beat egg substitute, flour, and evaporated milk until smooth. Pour over top and bake about 45 minutes in 350°F (180°C, or gas mark 4) oven.

—
3 servings

Each with: 397 Calories (26% from Fat, 50% from Protein, 24% from Carb); 48 g Protein; 11 g Total Fat; 6 g Unsaturated Fat; 3 g Monounsaturated Fat; 2 g Polyunsaturated Fat; 23 g Carb; 1 g Fiber; 16 g Sugar; 918 mg Phosphorus; 913 mg Calcium; 1144 mg Sodium; 838 mg Potassium; 1105 IU Vitamin A; 224 mg ATE Vitamin E; 15 mg Vitamin C; 30 mg Cholesterol

Not Exactly Eggs Benedict

This will remind you of Eggs Benedict, but it's easier to fix. Eggs are baked in cheese until well enough done, then served on English muffins in a breakfast that is filling as well as tasty.

½ cup (115 g) low fat cheddar cheese, shredded

4 eggs

¼ cup (60 g) fat-free sour cream

3 tablespoons (45 ml) skim milk

½ teaspoon prepared mustard

⅛ teaspoon black pepper

¼ teaspoon Worcestershire sauce

1½ tablespoons (12 g) all purpose flour

2 English muffins, split and toasted

Sprinkle half the cheese evenly over the bottom of greased baking dish. Break and slip eggs onto cheese in dish. Beat together remaining ingredients except remaining cheese and muffins. Pour over eggs, sprinkle with remaining cheese. Bake in a 325°F (170°C, or gas mark 3) oven until whites are set and yolks are soft and creamy, about 25 to 30 minutes. Serve over toasted muffin halves.

—
2 servings

Each with: 412 Calories (41% from Fat, 29% from Protein, 30% from Carb); 29 g Protein; 19 g Total Fat; 7 g Unsaturated Fat; 6 g Monounsaturated Fat; 2 g Polyunsaturated Fat; 30 g Carb; 2 g Fiber; 3 g Sugar; 512 mg Phosphorus; 363 mg Calcium; 659 mg Sodium; 342 mg Potassium; 795 IU Vitamin A; 225 mg ATE Vitamin E; 2 mg Vitamin C; 510 mg Cholesterol

Fancy Baked Egg Scramble

Here's a great company breakfast that no one will suspect is low calorie and full of nutrition (unless you want to brag about it of course). Eggs and vegetables are baked in a cheesy, creamy sauce with a crunchy topping that really makes this something special.

EGGS

2 tablespoons (28 g) unsalted butter

¼ cup (40 g) onion, chopped

¼ cup (38 g) green bell pepper, chopped

2 cups (300 g) ham, cubed

3 cups (700 ml) egg substitute

8 ounces (225 g) mushrooms, sliced

SAUCE

2 tablespoons (16 g) all purpose flour

1 tablespoon (14 g) unsalted butter

1½ cups (355 ml) skim milk

2 ounces (55 g) Swiss cheese, shredded

¼ cup (25 g) Parmesan cheese, grated

TOPPING

1 cup (115 g) bread crumbs

¼ cup (25 g) Parmesan cheese, grated

2 tablespoons (8 g) fresh parsley, chopped

Preheat oven to 350°F (180°C, or gas mark 4). Grease a 2-quart (1.9 L) baking dish. Melt 2 tablespoons (28 g) butter in large skillet. Cook and stir onion and green bell pepper until onion is crisp-tender. Add ham and egg substitute; cook over medium heat until eggs are firm but moist, stirring occasionally. Fold in mushrooms. Remove from heat. Melt 1 tablespoon (14 g) butter in medium saucepan. Blend in flour; cook until smooth and bubbly. Gradually add skim milk; cook until mixture boils and thickens, stirring constantly. Add Swiss cheese and ¼ cup (25 g) Parmesan cheese; stir until smooth. Fold scrambled eggs into sauce. Pour into greased pan. Combine all topping ingredients and sprinkle over eggs. Bake at 350°F (180°C, or gas mark 4) for 25 to 30 minutes or until light golden brown.

---

6 servings

Each with: 424 Calories (43% from Fat, 36% from Protein, 21% from Carb); 37 g Protein; 20 g Total Fat; 9 g Unsaturated Fat; 6 g Monounsaturated Fat; 3 g Polyunsaturated Fat; 22 g Carb; 2 g Fiber; 3 g Sugar; 512 mg Phosphorus; 381 mg Calcium; 1021 mg Sodium; 897 mg Potassium; 996 IU Vitamin A; 115 mg ATE Vitamin E; 9 mg Vitamin C; 53 mg Cholesterol

Fiesta Eggs

Green chilies and taco seasoning provide the Southwestern flavor of this beef, egg, and cheese bake. It's as good for lunch and dinner as breakfast, but that is when we usually have it.

½ pound (225 g) extra lean ground beef

2 tablespoons (6 g) taco seasoning mix

¾ cup (86 g) low fat Monterey Jack cheese, shredded

1 cup (115 g) low fat cheddar cheese, shredded

4 ounces (115 g) green chilies, diced

1½ cups (355 ml) skim milk

⅓ cup (42 g) all purpose flour

2 cups (475 ml) egg substitute

½ cup (130 g) salsa

In medium skillet, brown ground beef; drain off excess fat. Stir in taco seasoning mix. In 12 × 8-inch (30 × 20 cm) baking dish, toss beef mixture with cheese and chilies. In large bowl, blend a small amount of skim milk into flour until smooth. Stir in remaining skim milk and egg substitute. Pour milk mixture over mixture in dish. Bake at 350°F (180°C, or gas mark 4) for 40 to 50 minutes or until knife inserted in center comes out clean. Let stand 10 minutes before cutting into serving pieces. Spoon salsa over servings.

—
4 servings

Each with: 429 Calories (39% from Fat, 43% from Protein, 17% from Carb); 45 g Protein; 18 g Total Fat; 7 g Unsaturated Fat; 7 g Monounsaturated Fat; 3 g Polyunsaturated Fat; 18 g Carb; 1 g Fiber; 2 g Sugar; 637 mg Phosphorus; 464 mg Calcium; 921 mg Sodium; 893 mg Potassium; 1011 IU Vitamin A; 91 mg ATE Vitamin E; 15 mg Vitamin C; 54 mg Cholesterol

Breakfast in a Pocket

This breakfast sandwich starts with hard boiled eggs so it's really quick to make if you have the eggs cooked ahead of time. We then add cheese and vegetables to up the nutrition level, ending up with a filling meal for around 350 calories.

3 eggs, hard boiled

2 ounces (55 g) low fat cheddar cheese, grated

2 whole wheat pita breads, 6-inch (15 cm)

1 cup (180 g) tomato, chopped

½ cup (52 g) sprouts

Peel and slice hard boiled eggs. Grate cheese. Divide cheese and egg between pocket bread halves and microwave approximately 25 seconds or until cheese is melted. Add tomato and sprouts.

—
2 servings

Each with: 358 Calories (29% from Fat, 28% from Protein, 43% from Carb); 24 g Protein; 12 g Total Fat; 4 g Unsaturated Fat; 4 g Monounsaturated Fat; 2 g Polyunsaturated Fat; 38 g Carb; 2 g Fiber; 4 g Sugar; 385 mg Phosphorus; 225 mg Calcium; 621 mg Sodium; 390 mg Potassium; 1116 IU Vitamin A; 138 mg ATE Vitamin E; 10 mg Vitamin C; 374 mg Cholesterol

Baked French Toast

This makes an easy make-ahead breakfast for a weekend or holiday.

8 slices whole wheat bread, cubed

¾ cup (175 ml) egg substitute

3 tablespoons (27 g) sugar

1 teaspoon vanilla

2¼ cups (535 ml) skim milk

¼ cup (31 g) all purpose flour

6 tablespoons (6 g) brown sugar substitute, such as Splenda

½ teaspoon cinnamon, packed

2 tablespoons (28 g) unsalted butter

2 cups blueberries, fresh (290 g) or frozen (310 g)

Cut bread into cubes and place in a greased 9 × 13-inch (23 × 33 cm) baking dish. In a medium bowl, lightly beat egg substitute, sugar, and vanilla. Stir in the skim milk until well blended. Pour over bread, turning pieces to coat well. Cover and refrigerate overnight. Preheat oven to 375°F (190°C, or gas mark 5). In a small bowl, combine the flour, brown sugar substitute, and cinnamon. Cut in butter until mixture resembles coarse crumbs. Turn bread over in baking dish. Cover with blueberries. Sprinkle evenly with crumb mixture. Bake about 40 minutes until golden brown.

—

6 servings

Each with: 391 Calories (16% from Fat, 12% from Protein, 71% from Carb); 12 g Protein; 7 g Total Fat; 3 g Saturated Fat; 2 g Monounsaturated Fat; 1 g Polyunsaturated Fat; 70 g Carb; 3 g Fiber; 39 g Sugar; 202 mg Phosphorus; 217 mg Calcium; 131 mg Sodium; 416 mg Potassium; 450 IU Vitamin A; 88 mg ATE Vitamin E; 2 mg Vitamin C; 13 mg Cholesterol

TIP:

You can substitute strawberries or raspberries or use some combination of fruit, if you prefer.

Strawberry Dream Pancakes

These taste and look like they contain a lot of calories, but they don't. Thanks to fat-free ingredients, the creamy rich topping contributes well under 100 calories. The strawberries up the nutrition, as does the whole wheat flour, providing a satisfying breakfast that doesn't look like diet food.

TOPPING

4½ ounces (130 g) fat-free frozen whipped topping, thawed

⅓ cup (77 g) fat-free sour cream

16 ounces (455 g) frozen strawberries, thawed

PANCAKES

2 cups (240 g) whole wheat pastry flour

¼ cup (50 g) sugar

2 tablespoons baking powder

½ teaspoon baking soda

½ cup (120 ml) egg substitute

1½, cups (355 ml) skim milk

8 ounces (225 g) fat-free sour cream

2 tablespoons (28 ml) canola oil

Thoroughly drain strawberries. Chop ½ cup (64 g) drained strawberries; reserve remainder for topping. Combine reserved strawberries, whipped topping, and ⅓ cup (77 g) sour cream. Set aside. In a medium bowl, mix flour, sugar, baking powder, and baking soda. In another medium bowl, mix egg substitute, skim milk, sour cream, and oil. Add to flour mixture. Add ½ cup (64 g) chopped strawberries. Stir only until combined; the batter will still be lumpy. Preheat griddle. Brush preheated griddle with oil. Using ¼ cup (55 g) batter for each pancake, cook over medium-high heat 2 to 3 minutes or until underside is golden brown and surface is bubbly. Turn and cook 2 to 3 minutes more or until other side is golden brown. Keep warm. Place a pancake on each of 6 serving plates. Spread with about ⅓ cup (85 g) of topping. Place remaining pancakes on top. Garnish with an additional dollop of topping and a fresh strawberry if desired.

—
6 servings

Each with: 389 Calories (34% from Fat, 12% from Protein, 54% from Carb); 13 g Protein; 15 g Total Fat; 7 g Unsaturated Fat; 5 g Monounsaturated Fat; 2 g Polyunsaturated Fat; 55 g Carb; 6 g Fiber; 20 g Sugar; 409 mg Phosphorus; 452 mg Calcium; 694 mg Sodium; 531 mg Potassium; 419 IU Vitamin A; 89 mg ATE Vitamin E; 45 mg Vitamin C; 22 mg Cholesterol

Strawberry Banana Three Ways Breakfast

If you are a strawberry and banana fan, this is the breakfast for you. Start with strawberry-banana muffins. But make them healthier by using whole wheat flour and holding down the amount of oil. Then don't make the huge muffins you think you need to fill you up. Instead, fill up on fresh strawberries and bananas topped with—what else—strawberry-banana yogurt.

MUFFINS

¾ cup (90 g) whole wheat pastry flour

2 tablespoons (3 g) sugar substitute, uch as Splenda

¼ cup (29 g) wheat germ

1¼ teaspoon baking powder

¼ teaspoon baking soda

2 tablespoons (28 ml) egg substitute

½ cup (120 ml) skim milk

¼ cup (60 ml) canola oil

½ cup (113 g) banana, mashed

½ cup (75 g) strawberries, chopped

FRUIT

4 cups (580 g) strawberries

3 cups (450 g) banana, sliced

8 ounces (225 g) low fat strawberry-banana yogurt

Stir together the dry ingredients. Mix together the rest of the ingredients and stir into dry, stirring until just moistened. Spoon into 6 greased or paper lined muffin tins. Bake at 350°F (180°C, or gas mark 4) for 20 to 25 minutes or until done. While muffins are baking, slice fruit into a bowl and top with yogurt.

—
6 servings

Each with: 352 Calories (27% from Fat, 9% from Protein, 64% from Carb); 8 g Protein; 11 g Total Fat; 1 g Saturated Fat; 6 g Monounsaturated Fat; 3 g Polyunsaturated Fat; 60 g Carb; 8 g Fiber; 28 g Sugar; 246 mg Phosphorus; 168 mg Calcium; 198 mg Sodium; 877 mg Potassium; 177 IU Vitamin A; 13 mg ATE Vitamin E; 79 mg Vitamin C; 4 mg Cholesterol

Stuffed Cantaloupe

Well it IS stuffed, but it's stuffed with fruit, not the usual kind of stuffing. This raises the question of how anything that tastes this good can have so much nutrition and be this low in calories. The answer of course is that's exactly why fruit is so good for us.

2 cantaloupes, halved and cleaned

16 ounces (455 g) strawberries, cleaned and halved

16 ounces (455 g) seedless green grapes

2 bananas, sliced

4 apricots, pitted and chopped in quarters

12 ounces (340 g) low fat blackberry yogurt

1 cup (125 g) granola

fresh mint, for garnish

Mix all fruit except cantaloupe. Heap everything into the cantaloupe center, spoon yogurt on top of fruit mixture, top with granola, and garnish with sprig of mint.

—
4 servings

Each with: 363 Calories (6% from Fat, 7% from Protein, 86% from Carb); 7 g Protein; 3 g Total Fat; 1 g Unsaturated Fat; 1 g Monounsaturated Fat; 0 g Polyunsaturated Fat; 84 g Carb; 7 g Fiber; 59 g Sugar; 199 mg Phosphorus; 167 mg Calcium; 129 mg Sodium; 920 mg Potassium; 855 IU Vitamin A; 9 mg ATE Vitamin E; 60 mg Vitamin C; 4 mg Cholesterol

Cherry Parfait

This is really more like a dessert than a breakfast, with sweet cherries added into a creamy mixture that is layered with shredded wheat cereal for crunch (and fiber).

1½ cups (233 g) cherries, pitted and cut into halves

½ cup (115 g) plain low fat yogurt

1 teaspoon honey

½ teaspoon vanilla extract

1 cup (49 g) shredded wheat, crumbled

In a bowl, combine the first 4 ingredients, mixing until blended. Layer into parfait glasses with cereal.

—
2 servings

Each with: 379 Calories (4% from Fat, 8% from Protein, 87% from Carb); 9 g Protein; 2 g Total Fat; 1 g Unsaturated Fat; 0 g Monounsaturated Fat; 0 g Polyunsaturated Fat; 90 g Carb; 10 g Fiber; 65 g Sugar; 229 mg Phosphorus; 169 mg Calcium; 58 mg Sodium; 1365 mg Potassium; 3545 IU Vitamin A; 9 mg ATE Vitamin E; 1 mg Vitamin C; 4 mg Cholesterol

Breakfast in Paradise Smoothies

This smoothie will whisk you away to the islands, with its bananas, melons, and papaya. Smoothies make a great quick breakfast, but if you aren't careful when building them, you'll be hungry again before noon. This one solves that problem with a generous amount of fruit and a boost from tofu for added protein.

8 ounces (225 g) soft tofu

2 cups (280 g) papaya, peeled and chopped

2 cups (300 g) banana, sliced

1 cup (160 g) cantaloupe, peeled and cubed

½ cup (120 ml) skim milk

½ cup (120 ml) orange juice

Place all ingredients in blender and process until smooth.

—

2 servings

Each with: 400 Calories (9% from Fat, 12% from Protein, 79% from Carb); 12 g Protein; 4 g Total Fat; 1 g Saturated Fat; 1 g Monounsaturated Fat; 2 g Polyunsaturated Fat; 85 g Carb; 9 g Fiber; 44 g Sugar; 216 mg Phosphorus; 182 mg Calcium; 63 mg Sodium; 1836 mg Potassium; 4842 IU Vitamin A; 38 mg ATE Vitamin E; 160 mg Vitamin C; 1 mg Cholesterol

Dreamcicle Smoothie

Low fat buttermilk and orange juice concentrate provide the flavor here as well as the nutrition. Oat bran gives it a nice fiber boost.

1 cup (235 ml) low fat buttermilk

⅓ cup (95 g) orange juice concentrate

2 tablespoons (30 g) brown sugar

1 teaspoon vanilla

¼ cup (24 g) oat bran

½ cup (115 g) crushed ice

In a blender container, combine low fat buttermilk, orange juice concentrate, brown sugar, vanilla, and oat bran. Cover and blend until smooth. With blender running, add ice slowly through the opening in lid. Blend until smooth and frothy.

—

1 serving

Each with: 407 Calories (6% from Fat, 12% from Protein, 82% from Carb); 12 g Protein; 3 g Total Fat; 1 g Saturated Fat; 1 g Monounsaturated Fat; 0 g Polyunsaturated Fat; 84 g Carb; 2 g Fiber; 76 g Sugar; 337 mg Phosphorus; 364 mg Calcium; 4 mg Iron; 317 mg Sodium; 1159 mg Potassium; 532 IU Vitamin A; 50 mg ATE Vitamin E; 134 mg Vitamin C; 10 mg Cholesterol

Mixed Fruit Smoothie

Smoothies make a quick and easy breakfast, and they are packed with nutrition. The protein from the yogurt will help to keep you from being hungry as the morning goes on.

2 cups (460 g) low fat peach yogurt

1 cup (145 g) blueberries

2 cups (300 g) banana, sliced

Mix all ingredients in a blender and then serve.

—

2 servings

Each with: 382 Calories (3% from Fat, 11% from Protein, 86% from Carb); 14 g Protein; 1 g Total Fat; 1 g Saturated Fat; 0 g Monounsaturated Fat; 0 g Polyunsaturated Fat; 108 g Carb; 8 g Fiber; 81 g Sugar; 350 mg Phosphorus; 388 mg Calcium; 145 mg Sodium; 1337 mg Potassium; 213 IU Vitamin A; 5 mg ATE Vitamin E; 28 mg Vitamin C; 5 mg Cholesterol

Full of Fruit Healthy Shake

This smoothie is quick to fix and eat, but it provides a huge amount of nutrients like antioxidants, as well as the bulk and protein to keep you from being hungry before lunch.

2 bananas

1 cup (160 g) cantaloupe

1 cup (145 g) blueberries

2 cups (460 g) nonfat vanilla yogurt

Place all of the ingredients into blender and blend until smooth. Thaw fruit if frozen.

—

2 servings

Each with: 413 Calories (8% from Fat, 14% from Protein, 78% from Carb); 15 g Protein; 4 g Total Fat; 2 g Unsaturated Fat; 1 g Monounsaturated Fat; 0 g Polyunsaturated Fat; 86 g Carb; 6 g Fiber; 66 g Sugar; 386 mg Phosphorus; 439 mg Calcium; 178 mg Sodium; 1366 mg Potassium; 3234 IU Vitamin A; 29 mg ATE Vitamin E; 55 mg Vitamin C; 12 mg Cholesterol

Lunches and Light Meals

These meals are equally good for lunch or dinner, but they represent a little lighter fare than some of the ones in following chapters. Most are around our 400-calorie target for a meal, but there are a few that are quite a bit lower than that. There are lots of meal salads here, full of vegetables that help to fill you, combined with lean meat or grains to make them even more substantial. There also are sandwiches and wraps and a few meal in a bowl kind of things. We particularly like these kinds of meals in warm weather, when you tend to want something cooler and lighter, but there are things here that are good year round.

Antipasto Supper Salad

We usually have a salad dinner at least once a week, especially during the summer when fresh, locally grown vegetables are available. This meal on a plate antipasto salad has a great assortment of vegetables, with a tomato-based sauce that eliminates the need for any additional salad dressing.

½ cup (120 ml) white vinegar

2 tablespoons (28 ml) olive oil

3 ounces (85 g) no-salt-added tomato paste

4 ounces (115 g) pimento

10 ounces (280 g) frozen green beans, cooked and cooled

1 cup (122 g) carrot, sliced

¼ cup (25 g) green olives, sliced

8 ounces (225 g) mushrooms, sliced

1 cup (160 g) red onion, sliced

24 cherry tomatoes

1½ cups (180 g) zucchini, sliced

2 cups (480 g) garbanzo beans

8 ounces (225 g) roasted red pepper

9 cups (423 g) romaine lettuce, torn into bite-sized pieces

4 ounces (115 g) salami

12 ounces (340 g) tuna, water packed

6 tablespoons (30 g) Parmesan cheese, grated

Combine vinegar, olive oil, and tomato paste in a saucepan and heat over medium heat until hot and well combined. Remove and let cool. Cut vegetables into bite-sized pieces and add to the cooled mixture. Add garbanzo beans and stir to combine. Divide lettuce among serving plates and top with vegetable mixture, meat, and fish. Sprinkle with the Parmesan cheese.

—
6 servings

Each with: 393 Calories (31% from Fat, 28% from Protein, 41% from Carb); 29 g Protein; 14 g Total Fat; 3 g Saturated Fat; 7 g Monounsaturated Fat; 3 g Polyunsaturated Fat; 43 g Carb; 12 g Fiber; 10 g Sugar; 374 mg Phosphorus; 119 mg Calcium; 738 mg Sodium; 1436 mg Potassium; 10 218 IU Vitamin A; 4 mg ATE Vitamin E; 144 mg Vitamin C; 42 mg Cholesterol

Colorful Chickpea, Chicken, and Rice Salad

I really like the flavor of this salad, but perhaps that's because I enjoy the taste of cumin, which is the main spice in the dressing. I also like the color (not to mention the nutrition) of the multicolor peppers.

2 cups (480 g) chickpeas, cooked

2 cups (380 g) brown rice, cooked

2 cups (280 g) cooked chicken breast, diced

½ cup (75 g) red bell pepper, diced

½ cup (75 g) green bell pepper, diced

½ cup (75 g) yellow bell pepper, diced

¼ cup (25 g) green onion, sliced

1 teaspoon sesame oil

½ teaspoon ground cumin

2 tablespoons (28 ml) lemon juice

1 tablespoon (15 ml) olive oil

2 teaspoons sesame seeds, toasted

Toss together chickpeas, rice, chicken, red, green, and yellow bell pepper, and green onion in a large bowl. Whisk together the sesame oil, cumin, lemon juice, and olive oil. Toss with salad. Sprinkle toasted sesame seeds on top.

—
4 servings

Each with: 427 Calories (22% from Fat, 30% from Protein, 48% from Carb); 32 g Protein; 10 g Total Fat; 2 g Saturated Fat; 5 g Monounsaturated Fat; 3 g Polyunsaturated Fat; 51 g Carb; 8 g Fiber; 6 g Sugar; 365 mg Phosphorus; 89 mg Calcium; 62 mg Sodium; 654 mg Potassium; 848 IU Vitamin A; 4 mg ATE Vitamin E; 141 mg Vitamin C; 60 mg Cholesterol

Cool and Curried Rice Salad

This rice salad actually makes a great lunch or light dinner. You could also reduce the serving size and use it as a side dish. I prefer it with the Reduced Fat Italian Dressing from chapter 2, but feel free to try the others.

6 cups (1.2 kg) brown rice, cooked, cold

1 cup (164 g) frozen corn, cooked and cooled

1 cup (100 g) celery, thinly sliced

1 cup (150 g) green bell pepper, chopped

¼ cup (25 g) olives, sliced

1 cup (180 g) plum tomato, chopped

½ cup (90 g) red onion, minced

¼ cup (60 g) dill pickles, chopped

½ teaspoon black pepper, or to taste

¼ teaspoon curry powder

2 tablespoons (32 g) chutney

⅓ cup (85 g) dressing of your choice, see recipes in chapter 2

6 cups (432 g) iceberg lettuce, torn into bite-sized pieces

3 eggs, hard boiled

Combine first 9 ingredients. Stir curry powder and chutney into dressing; pour over salad. Toss lightly and chill until serving time. To serve, mound on lettuce. Garnish with slices of hard-boiled eggs.

—
6 servings

Each with: 391 Calories (27% from Fat, 10% from Protein, 63% from Carb); 10 g Protein; 12 g Total Fat; 2 g Saturated Fat; 3 g Monounsaturated Fat; 4 g Polyunsaturated Fat; 62 g Carb; 6 g Fiber; 7 g Sugar; 264 mg Phosphorus; 72 mg Calcium; 312 mg Sodium; 545 mg Potassium; 853 IU Vitamin A; 40 mg ATE Vitamin E; 29 mg Vitamin C; 123 mg Cholesterol

Fiesta Salad

Here's a simple but flavorful main dish salad. It's good for warmer evenings or for lunch.

2 tablespoons (28 ml) olive oil

¼ cup (60 ml) lime juice

2 tablespoons (28 ml) lemon juice

1 teaspoon garlic, minced

1 teaspoon ground cumin

½ teaspoon dried oregano

2 boneless skinless chicken breast

8 cups (376 g) romaine lettuce, torn into bite-sized pieces

16 cherry tomatoes, halved

2 avocados, peeled and sliced

¼ cup (28 g) Swiss cheese, shredded

1 cup (63 g) tortilla chips, crumbled

¼ cup (60 g) fat-free sour cream

½ cup (130 g) salsa

Combine first 6 ingredients in a plastic zipper bag. Add chicken breast and marinate at least two hours, turning occasionally. Grill or sauté chicken breast until no longer pink. Cut into ½-inch (1.3 cm) thick slices. Divide lettuce between plates. Top with tomatoes, avocado, and chicken. Sprinkle with cheese and tortilla chips. Combine sour cream and salsa and pour over top.

—

4 servings

Each with: 403 Calories (55% from Fat, 16% from Protein, 30% from Carb); 17 g Protein; 26 g Total Fat; 5 g Saturated Fat; 15 g Monounsaturated Fat; 4 g Polyunsaturated Fat; 31 g Carb; 11 g Fiber; 4 g Sugar; 278 mg Phosphorus; 195 mg Calcium; 366 mg Sodium; 1137 mg Potassium; 7384 IU Vitamin A; 20 mg ATE Vitamin E; 61 mg Vitamin C; 30 mg Cholesterol

French Style Bean Salad

This makes a great luncheon salad. It can also be a main dish and will provide plenty of nutrition and bulk to get you through the night. If you can't find cannellini beans, use great northern or navy beans.

2 cups (512 g) cannellini beans, drained and rinsed

13 ounces (365 g) tuna, drained

1 cup (180 g) tomato, seeded and diced

½ cup (80 g) red onion, chopped

2 tablespoons (28 ml) lemon juice

1 tablespoon (11 g) Dijon mustard

¼ cup (60 ml) olive oil

¼ cup (10 g) fresh basil, chopped

6 cups (432 g) iceberg lettuce, torn into bite-sized pieces

Combine beans, tuna, tomato, and onion in large bowl. Combine lemon juice and mustard in small bowl. Gradually whisk in olive oil. Add to salad. Mix in basil. Serve over lettuce.

—

4 servings

Each with: 375 Calories (40% from Fat, 32% from Protein, 27% from Carb); 31 g Protein; 17 g Total Fat; 3 g Saturated Fat; 11 g Monounsaturated Fat; 3 g Polyunsaturated Fat; 26 g Carb; 9 g Fiber; 4 g Sugar; 393 mg Phosphorus; 146 mg Calcium; 312 mg Sodium; 894 mg Potassium; 798 IU Vitamin A; 6 mg ATE Vitamin E; 15 mg Vitamin C; 39 mg Cholesterol

He Went to Paris (for This Nicoise Salad)

OK, so maybe the name of the recipe was influenced by seeing Jimmy Buffett in concert. (*He Went to Paris* is one of his songs for anyone that doesn't recognize the reference.) The ingredients in this salad are typical of the type of salad served in Nice, France.

1 ounce (28 g) anchovies, minced

2 teaspoons Dijon mustard

3 tablespoons (45 ml) red wine vinegar

2 tablespoons (28 ml) olive oil

4 cups (228 g) butter lettuce

1 can (5 ounces, or 140 g) tuna, drained

2 eggs, hard boiled, halved

1 large tomato, cut into wedges

2 medium potatoes, peeled, cooked, and sliced

½ cup (50 g) green beans, cooked, drained, and cooled

½ cup (75 g) green bell pepper, sliced and slivered

½ cup (80 g) red onion, cut in rounds

½ cup (85 g) black olives, drained

½ cup (35 g) mushrooms, thinly sliced

14 ounces (390 g) artichoke hearts, drained

½ cup (17 g) alfalfa sprouts

Combine first 4 ingredients to make dressing. Line a platter with butter lettuce. Place tuna in center. Arrange rest of ingredients in groups around tuna. Allow guest to choose their own ingredients for their salad or divide among 4 plates.

—
4 servings

Each with: 397 Calories (32% from Fat, 24% from Protein, 44% from Carb); 24 g Protein; 14 g Total Fat; 3 g Saturated Fat; 8 g Monounsaturated Fat; 2 g Polyunsaturated Fat; 45 g Carb; 10 g Fiber; 5 g Sugar; 385 mg Phosphorus; 126 mg Calcium; 567 mg Sodium; 1538 mg Potassium; 2391 IU Vitamin A; 44 mg ATE Vitamin E; 63 mg Vitamin C; 147 mg Cholesterol

Italian Dinner Salad

This is a meal on a plate. This may be only a salad, but I guarantee you won't walk away from the table hungry.

SALAD

4 cups (188 g) romaine lettuce, finely chopped

2 cups (180 g) cabbage, finely chopped

1 cup (150 g) green bell pepper, chopped

1 cup (150 g) red bell pepper, chopped

4 ounces (115 g) black olives

½ cup (50 g) celery, thinly sliced

2 cups (480 g) garbanzo beans, drained

4 ounces (115 g) dry salami, cut up

4 ounces (115 g) Swiss cheese, cut up

6 ounces (170 g) boneless chicken breast, cooked and chopped

DRESSING

¼ cup (60 ml) olive oil

2 tablespoons (28 ml) red wine vinegar

1 teaspoon balsamic vinegar

½ teaspoon garlic, minced

1 teaspoon lemon juice

1 tablespoon (11 g) Dijon mustard

1 teaspoon sugar

2 tablespoons (12 g) Italian seasoning

⅛ teaspoon black pepper, fresh ground

Divide lettuce between 6 plates. Arrange other vegetables, meats, and cheese over lettuce. Shake dressing ingredients together and drizzle over salads.

—

6 servings

Each with: 403 Calories (51% from Fat, 22% from Protein, 27% from Carb); 23 g Protein; 23 g Total Fat; 7 g Saturated Fat; 13 g Monounsaturated Fat; 2 g Polyunsaturated Fat; 28 g Carb; 7 g Fiber; 5 g Sugar; 313 mg Phosphorus; 282 mg Calcium; 846 mg Sodium; 611 mg Potassium; 3468 IU Vitamin A; 42 mg ATE Vitamin E; 91 mg Vitamin C; 52 mg Cholesterol

Meal on a Plate Chicken Caesar Salad

This is a pretty traditional chicken Caesar salad, except for the mushrooms, which I happened to like even before I found out they added bulk with almost no calories. This is a great quick meal when you don't feel like spending a long time cooking.

DRESSING

¼ cup (60 ml) olive oil

1 clove garlic, minced

1 tablespoon (15 ml) lemon juice

2 tablespoons (28 ml) red wine vinegar

½ teaspoon Worcestershire sauce

SALAD

1 pound (455 g) boneless chicken breasts

1 pound (455 g) romaine lettuce

8 ounces (225 g) mushrooms, sliced

1 cup (30 g) croutons

¼ cup (25 g) Parmesan cheese, grated

¼ teaspoon black pepper, fresh ground

Mix together dressing ingredients. Shake well in a jar with a tight fitting lid. Place ½ of dressing in a zipper baggie with chicken breasts and marinate several hours. Remove and discard dressing. Grill chicken until done. Slice into strips. Place lettuce on plates. Place mushrooms and chicken on top. Add croutons and sprinkle with cheese and black pepper. Serve with remaining dressing.

—

4 servings

Each with: 399 Calories (46% from Fat, 42% from Protein, 12% from Carb); 42 g Protein; 20 g Total Fat; 4 g Saturated Fat; 12 g Monounsaturated Fat; 3 g Polyunsaturated Fat; 12 g Carb; 3 g Fiber; 3 g Sugar; 397 mg Phosphorus; 133 mg Calcium; 250 mg Sodium; 785 mg Potassium; 6637 IU Vitamin A; 14 mg ATE Vitamin E; 31 mg Vitamin C; 102 mg Cholesterol

Mega Waldorf Salad with Chicken and Blue Cheese Dressing

The trouble with Waldorf salad is that it usually has more calories than you want in a side salad, but it isn't enough for a meal. We decided to attack the second part of the problem, adding more veggies and chicken breast to make it into a complete meal. Then to add a little more interest, we topped it with a tangy blue cheese dressing. Now it not only fills you like a full meal, but it has the taste that will keep you coming back.

¼ cup (60 ml) lime juice

¼ cup (60 g) low fat mayonnaise

2 ounces (55 g) blue cheese, crumbled

¼ cup (60 g) fat-free sour cream

4 boneless skinless chicken breast, cooked and cut into bite-sized pieces

4 granny smith apples, cored and chopped into bite-sized pieces

1 cup (122 g) carrot, sliced

1 cup (71 g) broccoli florets

1 cup (100 g) celery, sliced

½ cup (75 g) raisins

6 cups (342 g) lettuce, preferably red

2 ounces (55 g) walnuts, chopped and toasted

Squeeze juice from lime into medium bowl; add mayonnaise, cheese, and sour cream. Whisk until well blended (or blend in food processor or blender). Add remaining ingredients except lettuce and walnuts, stirring until coated with dressing. Divide lettuce among 4 plates, mound a quarter of the chicken mixture in middle of each plate, and top with a quarter of the walnuts.

—

4 servings

Each with: 414 Calories (34% from Fat, 24% from Protein, 42% from Carb); 26 g Protein; 16 g Total Fat; 5 g Saturated Fat; 4 g Monounsaturated Fat; 6 g Polyunsaturated Fat; 46 g Carb; 7 g Fiber; 31 g Sugar; 372 mg Phosphorus; 175 mg Calcium; 434 mg Sodium; 981 mg Potassium; 4654 IU Vitamin A; 47 mg ATE Vitamin E; 37 mg Vitamin C; 59 mg Cholesterol

More than the Usual Shrimp Remoulade

Shrimp remoulade is a dish of French origin that is often found on luncheon menus and typically consists of just lettuce, shrimp, and the remoulade sauce. Here we add more vegetables to make it a more complete meal. It's perfect for lunch or a summer evening dinner.

¼ cup (44 g) mustard, Creole or Dijon

2 tablespoons (14 g) paprika

1 teaspoon cayenne pepper

½ cup (120 ml) tarragon vinegar

⅓ cup (60 ml) olive oil

1½ cups (150 g) scallions, coarsely chopped

½ cup (50 g) celery, finely chopped

½ cup (30 g) fresh parsley, coarsely chopped

3 pounds (1⅓ kg) shrimp

1 large iceberg lettuce, trimmed and cut into ¼-inch (6 mm) wide shred

8 ounces (225 g) mushrooms, sliced

1 cup (110 g) carrot, shredded

1 cup (120 g) zucchini, shredded

1 cup (150 g) red bell pepper, finely chopped

To prepare the remoulade sauce, combine the mustard, paprika, and cayenne pepper in a deep bowl and stir with a wire whisk until all the ingredients are thoroughly combined. Beat in the vinegar. Then, whisking constantly, pour in the oil in a slow, thin stream and continue to beat until the sauce is smooth and thick. Add the scallions, celery, and parsley and mix well. Cover the bowl tightly with plastic wrap and let the sauce rest at room temperature for at least 4 hours before serving. Meanwhile, shell the shrimp. Bring 2 quarts (1.9 L) of water to a simmer, drop in the shrimp and cook, uncovered, for 3 to 5 minutes, until the shrimp are pink and firm. With a slotted spoon, transfer the shrimp to a plate to cool. Then chill them until ready to serve. Just before serving, mound the shredded lettuce on 8 chilled individual serving plates, add the mushrooms, carrot, zucchini, and red bell pepper, and arrange the shrimp on top. Spoon the remoulade sauce over the shrimp and serve at once.

—
8 servings

Each with: 312 Calories (37% from Fat, 48% from Protein, 15% from Carb); 38 g Protein; 13 g Total Fat; 2 g Unsaturated Fat; 7 g Monounsaturated Fat; 2 g Polyunsaturated Fat; 12 g Carb; 4 g Fiber; 6 g Sugar; 429 mg Phosphorus; 148 mg Calcium; 287 mg Sodium; 844 mg Potassium; 4694 IU Vitamin A; 92 mg ATE Vitamin E; 57 mg Vitamin C; 259 mg Cholesterol

Hot Chinese Chicken Salad

In some ways, this is more like fried rice than a salad. But we've come to really like the addition of wilted lettuce to Chinese dishes. And this one gives you lots of things to like, from crispy chicken to vegetables, all for fewer than 350 calories.

6 boneless skinless chicken breasts, cut up

3 tablespoons (24 g) cornstarch

3 tablespoons (45 ml) canola oil

⅛ teaspoon garlic powder

8 ounces (225 g) sliced mushrooms

1 cup (100 g) celery, sliced diagonally

1 cup (160 g) onion, chopped

1 cup (110 g) carrot, shredded

1 cup (180 g) fresh tomato, cut in chunks

1 cup (124 g) water chestnuts, sliced

¼ cup (60 ml) low sodium soy sauce

3 cups (216 g) iceberg lettuce, shredded

3 cups (576 g) brown rice, cooked

Roll or shake chicken in cornstarch. Heat oil in large fry pan or wok at medium-high. Cook chicken 15 to 20 minutes in oil. Sprinkle with garlic powder while cooking. Add all vegetables. Stir. Stir in soy sauce. Cover and reduce heat. Simmer 5 minutes. Add lettuce. Remove from heat, toss, and serve at once with rice.

6 servings

Each with: 327 Calories (24% from Fat, 26% from Protein, 49% from Carb); 22 g Protein; 9 g Total Fat; 1 g Unsaturated Fat; 5 g Monounsaturated Fat; 3 g Polyunsaturated Fat; 41 g Carb; 5 g Fiber; 6 g Sugar; 303 mg Phosphorus; 52 mg Calcium; 441 mg Sodium; 777 mg Potassium; 2968 IU Vitamin A; 4 mg ATE Vitamin E; 10 mg Vitamin C; 41 mg Cholesterol

Chicken Kabobs with Chickpea Salad

It's kind of hard to say where this dish gets its flavor from (maybe I just need to travel more). But to me it seems Middle Eastern or possibly Indian. Chicken breasts kabobs are marinated in a yogurt sauce similar to tandoori chicken and then grilled and served over a salad featuring chickpeas and onion for a delightful taste sensation as well as great fiber and nutrient content.

1 cup (230 g) plain yogurt

½ teaspoon garlic, finely chopped

½ teaspoon ground cumin

½ teaspoon black pepper, divided

1 pound (455 g) boneless skinless chicken breast, cut in 1-inch (2.5 cm) cubes

2 cups (480 g) chickpeas, rinsed and drained

½ cup (90 g) red onion, thinly sliced

¼ cup (25 g) celery, sliced

1 cup (60 g) fresh parsley

2 tablespoons (28 ml) olive oil

2 teaspoons red wine vinegar

Heat grill to medium-high. In a shallow baking dish, combine the yogurt, garlic, cumin, and ¼ teaspoon black pepper. Thread the chicken onto 8 skewers and set them in the yogurt marinade, turning to coat. Refrigerate at least 10 minutes or as much as overnight. Meanwhile, in a large bowl, combine the chickpeas, onion, celery, parsley, oil, vinegar, and ¼ teaspoon black pepper. Remove the chicken from the marinade and cook on a well-oiled grill, turning occasionally, until cooked through, about 10 minutes. Divide the chickpea salad among plates and serve with the chicken.

—
4 servings

Each with: 397 Calories (25% from Fat, 37% from Protein, 38% from Carb); 37 g Protein; 11 g Total Fat; 2 g Unsaturated Fat; 6 g Monounsaturated Fat; 2 g Polyunsaturated Fat; 38 g Carb; 7 g Fiber; 17 g Sugar; 445 mg Phosphorus; 170 mg Calcium; 128 mg Sodium; 779 mg Potassium; 1371 IU Vitamin A; 14 mg ATE Vitamin E; 24 mg Vitamin C; 69 mg Cholesterol

Italian Veggie Noodles

This is kind of a poor man's lasagna. It's quick to throw together for lunch or dinner but full of veggies and nutrition.

8 ounces (225 g) whole wheat noodles, uncooked

1½ cups (375 g) low fat ricotta cheese

2 cups (240 g) zucchini, chopped

1 cup (150 g) red bell pepper, diced

2 cups (140 g) mushrooms chopped

½ cup (20 g) fresh herbs, chives, basil, and parsley

Cook noodles. Drain and return to pot. Add other ingredients and cook for 5 to 7 minutes until warmed.

—
4 servings

Each with: 357 Calories (20% from Fat, 23% from Protein, 57% from Carb); 21 g Protein; 9 g Total Fat; 5 g Unsaturated Fat; 2 g Monounsaturated Fat; 1 g Polyunsaturated Fat; 54 g Carb; 3 g Fiber; 4 g Sugar; 383 mg Phosphorus; 306 mg Calcium; 129 mg Sodium; 617 mg Potassium; 1873 IU Vitamin A; 97 mg ATE Vitamin E; 90 mg Vitamin C; 29 mg Cholesterol

Thai Noodle Bowl

This is a healthy version of the noodle bowls that have become so popular. Flavored with peanut butter, lime juice, and garlic, it will satisfy the taste buds without excess calories.

4 ounces (115 g) whole wheat spaghetti

2 tablespoons (32 g) peanut butter

3 tablespoons (45 ml) lime juice

1 teaspoon garlic, minced

1 teaspoon fresh ginger, peeled and grated

½ cup (75 g) edamame

10 ounces (280 g) frozen stir-fry vegetables

2 tablespoons (18 g) chopped peanuts

¼ cup (25 g) scallions, sliced

Cook pasta according to directions. In a skillet, sauté peanut butter, lime juice, garlic, and ginger for 1 minute. Add edamame and vegetables and cook for 12 minutes until vegetables are tender; pour over pasta. Top with peanuts and scallions.

—
2 servings

Each with: 411 Calories (21% from Fat, 16% from Protein, 63% from Carb); 18 g Protein; 11 g Total Fat; 2 g Unsaturated Fat; 4 g Monounsaturated Fat; 3 g Polyunsaturated Fat; 70 g Carb; 12 g Fiber; 2 g Sugar; 299 mg Phosphorus; 82 mg Calcium; 106 mg Sodium; 627 mg Potassium; 7336 IU Vitamin A; 0 mg ATE Vitamin E; 24 mg Vitamin C; 0 mg Cholesterol

Better BLT

Make your BLT healthier by stacking the tomato thickly and serving with fruit on the side for extra nutrition.

8 slices low sodium bacon

2 tablespoons (28 g) low fat mayonnaise

4 slices whole wheat bread, toasted

4 leaves romaine lettuce

1 large tomato, sliced

1 pear

Cook bacon. Spread mayonnaise on toast and top with bacon, lettuce, and tomato. Serve pear on the side.

—
2 servings

Each with: 412 Calories (35% from Fat, 18% from Protein, 47% from Carb); 18 g Protein; 16 g Total Fat; 5 g Unsaturated Fat; 7 g Monounsaturated Fat; 2 g Polyunsaturated Fat; 49 g Carb; 8 g Fiber; 18 g Sugar; 304 mg Phosphorus; 88 mg Calcium; 726 mg Sodium; 817 mg Potassium; 2454 IU Vitamin A; 4 mg ATE Vitamin E; 28 mg Vitamin C; 37 mg Cholesterol

Turkey and Avocado Wrap

This recipe features low calorie turkey, healthy avocado, high nutrient density spinach, and fresh fruit. How could you ask for a better low calorie lunch?

5 ounces (140 g) turkey breast, sliced

1 avocado, chopped

2 cups (60 g) spinach

2 whole wheat tortillas, 8-inch (20 cm)

2 nectarines or peaches

Wrap turkey, avocado, and spinach in tortilla. Serve nectarines or peaches on the side.

—
2 servings

Each with: 397 Calories (38% from Fat, 23% from Protein, 40% from Carb); 23 g Protein; 17 g Total Fat; 3 g Unsaturated Fat; 10 g Monounsaturated Fat; 3 g Polyunsaturated Fat; 41 g Carb; 10 g Fiber; 11 g Sugar; 281 mg Phosphorus; 70 mg Calcium; 228 mg Sodium; 1137 mg Potassium; 3392 IU Vitamin A; 0 mg ATE Vitamin E; 23 mg Vitamin C; 43 mg Cholesterol

Dinners: Chicken and Turkey

Chicken and turkey are naturals for our 400-calorie meals. They are naturally low in fat and calories. There are a couple of things to remember to help you make the best choices when having chicken or turkey. First is that much of the fat is in the skin, so you should avoid eating that. The second is that white meat is leaner than dark meat. In keeping with both of these suggestions, you'll find that many of these recipes call for boneless, skinless chicken breasts. These have the additional advantage that they can be used in a wide variety of recipes. This can easily be seen in this chapter as we have not only traditional food from the United States, but around the world, with recipes that came from Italy, Spain, Mexico, Greece, France, and a variety of Asian recipes. And that's just the beginning.

Honey Fried Chicken Dinner

Here's a complete fried chicken dinner for less than 400 calories. To make this possible, we oven fry lean chicken breasts, drizzled with a honey glaze, and then serve it with red potatoes and broccoli.

1 pound (455 g) boneless skinless chicken breast

2 tablespoons (22 g) Dijon mustard

4 tablespoons (28 g) dry bread crumbs

4 small red potatoes, quartered

2 teaspoons olive oil

4 cups (284 g) fresh broccoli florets

¼ cup (85 g) honey

2 tablespoons (28 ml) low sodium chicken broth, or water

Preheat oven to 450°F (230°C, or gas mark 8). Coat a large baking sheet with nonstick vegetable oil spray. Butterfly chicken by cutting each piece in half horizontally, almost through to the other side, but not completely. Open chicken breast half to make one thin piece. Brush Dijon mustard over both sides. Place seasoned bread crumbs in a shallow dish; add chicken breasts and turn to coat each side. Transfer chicken to prepared baking sheet and spray the chicken breasts with nonstick vegetable oil spray. Bake 8 to 10 minutes until chicken is cooked through. Meanwhile, place red potatoes in a microwave-safe container with a lid, add olive oil, and toss to coat potatoes. Cover and microwave on high for 5 minutes until potatoes are tender. Place broccoli in a microwave-safe container with a lid, cover, and microwave on high for 3 minutes until broccoli is crisp-tender. In a small bowl, whisk together honey and chicken broth. Transfer chicken to individual plates and drizzle honey mixture over top. Serve red potatoes and broccoli on the side.

—

4 servings

Each with: 395 Calories (11% from Fat, 33% from Protein, 56% from Carb); 33 g Protein; 5 g Total Fat; 1 g Unsaturated Fat; 2 g Monounsaturated Fat; 1 g Polyunsaturated Fat; 56 g Carb; 4 g Fiber; 20 g Sugar; 403 mg Phosphorus; 85 mg Calcium; 244 mg Sodium; 1402 mg Potassium; 2176 IU Vitamin A; 7 mg ATE Vitamin E; 104 mg Vitamin C; 66 mg Cholesterol

Really Low in Calories Chicken Shepherd's Pie

Shepherd's pie can be a high calorie, low nutrient dish, with its ground beef, buttery mashed potatoes, and cheese. So I went to work making a lower fat and calorie version for this book using chicken. And the problem I had was it was too LOW in calories. No matter how many veggies I added and how big the serving got, it just wasn't 400 calories. So you'll just have to content yourself with a 350-calorie mega meal.

2 tablespoons (16 g) cornstarch

1 cup (235 ml) low sodium chicken broth

3 cups (420 g) cooked chicken breast, diced

1 cup (150 g) red bell pepper, chopped

1 cup (160 g) red onion, chopped

20 ounces (570 g) frozen mixed vegetables

20 ounces (570 g) frozen broccoli

3 cups (610 g) mashed potatoes, prepared according to package directions

½ cup (58 g) low fat cheddar cheese, shredded

Mix cornstarch with broth. Heat until thickened and bubbly. Stir in chicken. Place in the bottom of a 9 × 9-inch (23 × 23 cm) baking dish. Cook vegetables until almost tender. Spread over chicken mixture. Cover with prepared mashed potatoes. Top with cheddar cheese. Heat under broiler until potatoes start to brown and cheese melts.

—
6 servings

Each with: 350 Calories (11% from Fat, 39% from Protein, 50% from Carb); 33 g Protein; 4 g Total Fat; 2 g Saturated Fat; 1 g Monounsaturated Fat; 1 g Polyunsaturated Fat; 43 g Carb; 9 g Fiber; 8 g Sugar; 377 mg Phosphorus; 145 mg Calcium; 809 mg Sodium; 916 mg Potassium; 5932 IU Vitamin A; 15 mg ATE Vitamin E; 96 mg Vitamin C; 64 mg Cholesterol

Chicken and Stuffing Bake

Creamed chicken and stuffing is served with broccoli for an every night Thanksgiving dinner. The use of chicken breasts and low fat soup holds down the fat content and the calories, providing a filling meal with fewer than 400 calories total.

6 ounces (170 g) stuffing mix

1½ pounds (680 g) boneless skinless chicken breast, cut in bite-sized pieces

1 can (10¾ ounces, or 305 g) low sodium cream of chicken soup

¼ cup (60 g) fat-free sour cream

16 ounces (455 g) frozen mixed vegetables, thawed

½ teaspoon black pepper

½ teaspoon garlic powder

½ teaspoon onion powder

4½ cup (320 g) broccoli florets, steamed until crisp-tender

Preheat oven to 400°F (200°C, or gas mark 6). Prepare stuffing according to package directions. Mix chicken, soup, sour cream, and vegetables. Place in a 13 × 9-inch (33 × 23 cm) baking pan and sprinkle with black pepper, onion powder, and garlic powder. Cover the chicken mixture with the stuffing. Bake 30 to 40 minutes or until chicken is done. Serve with broccoli.

—
6 servings

Each with: 361 Calories (17% from Fat, 39% from Protein, 44% from Carb); 35 g Protein; 7 g Total Fat; 2 g Unsaturated Fat; 2 g Monounsaturated Fat; 1 g Polyunsaturated Fat; 39 g Carb; 4 g Fiber; 5 g Sugar; 363 mg Phosphorus; 110 mg Calcium; 969 mg Sodium; 715 mg Potassium; 4985 IU Vitamin A; 38 mg ATE Vitamin E; 54 mg Vitamin C; 74 mg Cholesterol

Fit for Chicken à la King

Loaded with vegetables, this easy version of chicken à la king will satisfy your appetite and your taste buds.

8 ounces (225 g) whole wheat pasta

4 boneless skinless chicken breasts

2 cups (200 g) celery, chopped

1 cup (160 g) onion, chopped

2 cups (260 g) peas

1 cup (150 g) green bell pepper, chopped

2 cups (142 g) broccoli florets

1 can (10¾ ounces, or 305 g) low sodium cream of mushroom soup

Cook pasta according to package directions. Cut chicken breasts into small cubes and brown in a nonstick pan and set aside. Chop vegetables and sauté until they just start to turn soft. Add the mushroom soup and one can of water to the vegetables. Add the chicken and cook until chicken is done. Add the pasta and heat through.

—
4 servings

Each with: 356 Calories (9% from Fat, 30% from Protein, 61% from Carb); 27 g Protein; 4 g Total Fat; 1 g Unsaturated Fat; 1 g Monounsaturated Fat; 1 g Polyunsaturated Fat; 55 g Carb; 10 g Fiber; 8 g Sugar; 381 mg Phosphorus; 128 mg Calcium; 1116 mg Sodium; 1465 mg Potassium; 1281 IU Vitamin A; 12 mg ATE Vitamin E; 92 mg Vitamin C; 46 mg Cholesterol

Barbecue Chicken Dinner

Barbecued chicken is teamed with a rice pilaf full of vegetables for this quick and easy dinner.

4 boneless skinless chicken breasts

¼ cup (65 g) barbecue sauce

1 tablespoon (15 ml) olive oil

20 ounces (570 g) frozen mixed vegetables

2 cups (390 g) brown rice, cooked

4 tablespoons (28 g) sliced almonds

Grill chicken breast until chicken is done, about 8 minutes, brushing with barbecue sauce while cooking. Sauté vegetables in olive oil until tender, about 8 minutes. Add rice and heat until warm through. Top with almonds.

—
4 servings

Each with: 393 Calories (23% from Fat, 25% from Protein, 52% from Carb); 25 g Protein; 10 g Total Fat; 1 g Unsaturated Fat; 6 g Monounsaturated Fat; 2 g Polyunsaturated Fat; 51 g Carb; 9 g Fiber; 11 g Sugar; 330 mg Phosphorus; 73 mg Calcium; 250 mg Sodium; 560 mg Potassium; 6077 IU Vitamin A; 4 mg ATE Vitamin E; 5 mg Vitamin C; 41 mg Cholesterol

Stuffed Zucchini

This is perfect forwhen you don't get back to check the garden as often as you should and find a couple of zucchini that would make great softball bats. Discard the seeds and any center part of the squash that has gotten hard or stringy and put the rest of what you scoop out into the filling.

3 large zucchini

1¼ pounds (570 g) ground turkey

1 cup (160 g) onion, chopped

1 teaspoon garlic, crushed

2 cups (360 g) no-salt-added tomatoes

1½ cups (293 g) brown rice, cooked or (236 g) small whole wheat pasta

1 teaspoon dried basil

3 ounces (85 g) Swiss cheese, shredded

Cut the zucchini is half lengthwise. Scrape out the center, leaving a thickness of about a half inch (1.3 cm). Discard the seeds and chop the remainder. Cook the ground turkey, onion, and garlic in a large skillet until meat is done. Stir in tomatoes, rice or pasta, and basil. Cook the zucchini in boiling water until it begins to soften. Drain and place in baking pan. Divide the filling between the zucchini. Place a ½ ounce (15 g) of cheese on top of each. Place under broiler until cheese is melted and bubbly.

—
6 servings

Each with: 349 Calories (34% from Fat, 45% from Protein, 22% from Carb); 39 g Protein; 13 g Total Fat; 7 g Saturated Fat; 3 g Monounsaturated Fat; 2 g Polyunsaturated Fat; 19 g Carb; 2 g Fiber; 4 g Sugar; 329 mg Phosphorus; 332 mg Calcium; 148 mg Sodium; 732 mg Potassium; 824 IU Vitamin A; 17 mg Vitamin C; 98 mg Cholesterol

Go to Italy Tonight with Chicken Breast Cacciatore

This made a great tasting sauce with no extra work. And it's always nice to come home to a meal that's done and has filled the house with such an aroma. Paired with a broccoli and cauliflower combination, it also provides great nutrition.

1 cup (160 g) onion, sliced

6 boneless chicken breast

12 ounces (340 g) no-salt-added tomato paste

¼ teaspoon black pepper

½ teaspoon garlic powder

1 teaspoon dried oregano

1 teaspoon dried basil

¼ cup (60 ml) dry white wine

¼ cup (60 ml) water

4½ cups (320 g) broccoli florets, steamed until crisp-tender

4½ cups (450 g) cauliflower florets, steamed until crisp-tender

12 ounces (340 g) whole wheat pasta

Place onion in bottom of slow cooker. Place chicken on top. Combine remaining ingredients and pour over top. Cook on low for 8 to 10 hours. Serve with steamed broccoli and cauliflower and pasta cooked according to package directions.

—
6 servings

Each with: 385 Calories (6% from Fat, 31% from Protein, 64% from Carb); 31 g Protein; 3 g Total Fat; 1 g Saturated Fat; 0 g Monounsaturated Fat; 1 g Polyunsaturated Fat; 65 g Carb; 12 g Fiber; 10 g Sugar; 416 mg Phosphorus; 109 mg Calcium; 144 mg Sodium; 1275 mg Potassium; 1349 IU Vitamin A; 4 mg ATE Vitamin E; 115 mg Vitamin C; 42 mg Cholesterol

Pesto Chicken and Pasta

Pine nuts and fresh basil provide a pesto flavor to this flavorful dish, without the fat and sodium that canned pesto usually contains. The result is a healthier meal that's low in calories.

8 ounces (225 g) whole wheat pasta

1 teaspoon garlic, minced

30 cherry tomatoes, halved

2 cups (280 g) cooked chicken breast

1 tablespoon (15 ml) olive oil

½ cup (68 g) pine nuts

1 cup (40 g) chopped basil

Boil pasta according to directions. Sauté garlic, tomatoes, and chicken in olive oil for 3 to 5 minutes until warm. Add cooked pasta, pine nuts, and basil. Stir to combine and continue cooking for a few minutes longer until basil is limp.

—
4 servings

Each with: 378 Calories (42% from Fat, 30% from Protein, 29% from Carb); 29 g Protein; 18 g Total Fat; 2 g Unsaturated Fat; 7 g Monounsaturated Fat; 7 g Polyunsaturated Fat; 28 g Carb; 7 g Fiber; 1 g Sugar; 349 mg Phosphorus; 207 mg Calcium; 57 mg Sodium; 879 mg Potassium; 1602 IU Vitamin A; 4 mg ATE Vitamin E; 30 mg Vitamin C; 60 mg Cholesterol

Home-Style Italian Chicken Spaghetti Pie

Adding lots of chicken breast and vegetables and reducing the amount of pasta makes this one dish meal both satisfying and tasty.

8 ounces (225 g) whole wheat spaghetti, cooked

½ cup (120 ml) egg substitute

1 cup (225 g) fat-free cottage cheese

½ cup (80 g) onion, chopped

½ cup (75 g) green bell pepper, chopped

16 ounces (455 g) frozen Italian vegetable mix

2 cups (360 g) no-salt-added tomatoes, drained

1 teaspoon dried oregano

½ teaspoon garlic powder

3 cups (420 g) cooked chicken, cubed

¾ cup (83 g) part skim mozzarella, shredded

Cook spaghetti according to package directions. Drain. Mix in egg substitute. Form into a crust in a greased 10-inch (25 cm) pie pan. Top with cottage cheese. In a large skillet, cook onion and green bell pepper until tender. Add remaining ingredients except cheese and heat through. Spread over noodles and cottage cheese. Bake in 350°F (180°C, or gas mark 4) oven for 20 minutes. Sprinkle with mozzarella cheese about 5 minutes before the end of baking.

—

6 servings

Each with: 397 Calories (18% from Fat, 37% from Protein, 44% from Carb); 38 g Protein; 8 g Total Fat; 3 g Saturated Fat; 3 g Monounsaturated Fat; 2 g Polyunsaturated Fat; 45 g Carb; 7 g Fiber; 4 g Sugar; 446 mg Phosphorus; 244 mg Calcium; 232 mg Sodium; 724 mg Potassium; 4148 IU Vitamin A; 20 mg ATE Vitamin E; 30 mg Vitamin C; 62 mg Cholesterol

Mole Tostadas

Low fat chicken and black beans, simmered in a chocolate chili mole sauce, combine for the stuffing for these tostadas. Lettuce and fresh tomato add additional bulk and nutrition.

8 corn tortillas

1 teaspoon canola oil

1 cup (160 g) onion, chopped

½ teaspoon garlic, minced

1 tablespoon (6 g) cocoa powder

1 teaspoon chili powder

1 teaspoon ground cumin

½ teaspoon cinnamon

½ teaspoon sugar

½ teaspoon dried oregano

2 cups (360 g) no-salt-added tomatoes, drained

2 cups (344 g) black beans, rinsed and drained

2 cups (280 g) cooked chicken breast, shredded

2 cups (94 g) romaine lettuce, shredded

2 cups (360 g) tomato, chopped

Preheat oven to 425°F (220°C, or gas mark 7). Lightly spray large baking sheet with nonstick vegetable oil spray. Arrange tortillas in single layer on baking sheet and lightly spray them with nonstick vegetable oil spray. Bake until crisp, 6 to 8 minutes. Transfer tortillas to wire rack to cool. Meanwhile, heat oil in large nonstick skillet over medium heat. Add onion and garlic; cook, stirring frequently, until golden, about 7 minutes. Add cocoa, chili, cumin, cinnamon, sugar, and oregano; cook, stirring constantly, until fragrant, about 1 minute. Add tomatoes, beans, and chicken; bring to boil. Reduce heat and simmer, stirring occasionally, until thickened, 10 to 12 minutes. Spoon about ⅓ cup (85 g) of chili onto each tortilla. Top evenly with lettuce and tomato.

—
4 servings

Each with: 399 Calories (15% from Fat, 32% from Protein, 53% from Carb); 33 g Protein; 7 g Total Fat; 1 g Unsaturated Fat; 2 g Monounsaturated Fat; 2 g Polyunsaturated Fat; 54 g Carb; 11 g Fiber; 14 g Sugar; 546 mg Phosphorus; 190 mg Calcium; 1055 mg Sodium; 1428 mg Potassium; 2636 IU Vitamin A; 4 mg ATE Vitamin E; 39 mg Vitamin C; 60 mg Cholesterol

Classic Spanish Arroz Con Pollo, and Then Some

In this recipe, we've taken the classic Spanish chicken and rice dish and reduced the fat by using boneless skinless chicken breast and then added mushrooms and more vegetables than usual to make it even more filling without adding to the calories. Finally, we made it an easy to fix slow cooker recipe. If you prefer, you can still make it in a large covered skillet, following the same preparation steps, but simmer it in the skillet until the rice is tender, about 45 minutes, adding the peas and green bell pepper for the final 10 minutes.

1 tablespoon (15 ml) olive oil

2½ pounds (1.1 kg) boneless skinless chicken breast

1 cup (160 g) onion, finely chopped

6 ounces (170 g) mushrooms, sliced

1 teaspoon garlic, minced

¼ teaspoon black pepper

1½ cups (285 g) brown rice

¼ teaspoon saffron, or 1 teaspoon turmeric

2 cups (360 g) no-salt-added tomatoes

1½ cups (355 ml) low sodium chicken broth

½ cup (120 ml) white wine

¾ cups (113 g) green bell pepper, finely chopped

2 cups (260 g) frozen peas

In a nonstick skillet, heat oil over medium-high heat. Add chicken, in batches, and brown lightly on all sides. Transfer to slow cooker. Reduce heat to medium. Add onion and mushrooms and cook, stirring, until softened. Add garlic and black pepper and cook, stirring, for 1 minute. Add rice and stir until grains are well coated with mixture. Stir in saffron or turmeric, tomatoes, chicken broth, and white wine. Transfer to slow cooker and stir to combine with chicken. Cover and cook on low for 6 to 8 hours or on high for 3 to 4 hours until chicken is cooked through and rice is tender. Stir in green bell pepper and peas, cover, and cook on high for 20 minutes until vegetables are heated through.

—

6 servings

Each with: 384 Calories (14% from Fat, 55% from Protein, 30% from Carb); 51 g Protein; 6 g Total Fat; 1 g Saturated Fat; 3 g Monounsaturated Fat; 1 g Polyunsaturated Fat; 28 g Carb; 6 g Fiber; 7 g Sugar; 524 mg Phosphorus; 77 mg Calcium; 193 mg Sodium; 974 mg Potassium; 1332 IU Vitamin A; 11 mg ATE Vitamin E; 36 mg Vitamin C; 110 mg Cholesterol

TIP:

Feel free to substitute other chopped fresh vegetables, such as broccoli florets or bell peppers, for the tomatoes or cucumber.

Greek Mousaka

This variation of the typical Greek dish uses ground turkey rather than the more common lamb to hold down the fat. But the taste is still traditional, and it will definitely fill you up.

3 cups (700 ml) water

1½ pounds (680 g) eggplant, peeled and sliced

½ pound (225 g) ground turkey

1 cup (160 g) onion, chopped

2 teaspoons garlic, minced

½ teaspoon cinnamon

½ teaspoon dried oregano

1 cup (235 ml) low sodium chicken broth

⅔ cup (127 g) brown rice

8 ounces (225 g) no-salt-added tomato sauce

2 tablespoons unsalted butter

¼ cup (30 g) whole wheat pastry flour

1½ cups (355 ml) skim milk

½ cup (120 ml) egg substitute

¼ teaspoon nutmeg

Lightly grease a shallow 2-quart (1.9 L) baking dish. Bring 3 cups (700 ml) water to boil in a large nonstick skillet. Add eggplant, cover, reduce heat, and simmer 10 minutes or until tender. Remove to paper towels to drain. Wipe skillet. Add turkey, onion, and garlic. Cook until no longer pink. Stir in cinnamon and oregano, then broth and rice. Cover and simmer 10 minutes, stirring 2 or 3 times. Stir in tomato sauce. Remove from heat. Melt butter in a 2-quart (1.9 L) saucepan. Whisk in flour and cook, stirring 1 to 2 minutes, without letting mixture brown. Gradually whisk in skim milk. Cook, whisking constantly, 4 to 5 minutes until thickened and smooth. Whisk about ⅓ the hot mixture into beaten egg substitute and then whisk egg mixture into remaining sauce. Remove from heat; stir in nutmeg. Preheat oven to 350°F (180°C, or gas mark 4). To assemble, cover bottom of prepared baking dish with half the eggplant slices. Spoon on all the filling and then cover with remaining eggplant. Pour on topping. Bake 20 to 25 minutes or until hot and bubbly and top is lightly golden.

—
4 servings

Each with: 388 Calories (22% from Fat, 23% from Protein, 56% from Carb); 22 g Protein; 10 g Total Fat; 5 g Saturated Fat; 2 g Monounsaturated Fat; 2 g Polyunsaturated Fat; 55 g Carb; 9 g Fiber; 9 g Sugar; 355 mg Phosphorus; 220 mg Calcium; 451 mg Sodium; 1116 mg Potassium; 732 IU Vitamin A; 104 mg ATE Vitamin E; 12 mg Vitamin C; 37 mg Cholesterol

Cajun Chicken and Sausage Jambalaya

I love a good Jambalaya, but it is often not the best thing when you are trying to watch your calories. This one uses chicken and turkey sausage to hold down the fat level and includes more than the usual vegetables to add to the nutrition and that feeling of fullness.

1 pound (455 g) boneless chicken breast

4 cups (950 ml) water

2 cups (320 g) onion, chopped

1 cup (10 g) celery, sliced

1 tablespoon (10 g) garlic, minced

1 tablespoon (15 ml) olive oil

½ pound (225 g) turkey sausage

3 tablespoons (28 g) green bell pepper, chopped

¼ cup (25 g) green onion

2 cups (360 g) no-salt-added tomatoes

2 tablespoons (28 ml) Worcestershire sauce

¼ teaspoon dried thyme

¼ teaspoon cayenne pepper

1½ cups (285 g) brown rice

In a large saucepan, combine the chicken breasts, water, half the chopped onion, half the chopped celery, and one third of the garlic. Bring to a simmer over medium-high heat. Reduce the heat to medium-low and cook, partially covered, until the chicken juices run clear when pierced with a fork, 20 to 25 minutes. Remove the chicken breasts from the cooking liquid. In a sieve set over a large bowl, drain and reserve the cooking liquid. You should have about 4 cups (950 ml) of liquid; add water, if necessary. Chop the chicken breast meat coarsely and set it aside. Heat the oil in a 5-quart (4.7 L) Dutch oven. Add the sausage and cook over medium heat, stirring often, until lightly browned, about 5 minutes. Then stir in the remaining ingredients, breaking up the tomatoes with a spoon. Cook over medium-low heat, tightly covered, until the rice has absorbed all the liquid, about 45 minutes. Remove the Dutch oven from the heat, stir in the reserved chicken, cover, and let stand for 5 minutes.

—

6 servings

Each with: 416 Calories (25% from Fat, 28% from Protein, 47% from Carb); 29 g Protein; 12 g Total Fat; 4 g Saturated Fat; 4 g Monounsaturated Fat; 2 g Polyunsaturated Fat; 49 g Carb; 4 g Fiber; 6 g Sugar; 421 mg Phosphorus; 87 mg Calcium; 353 mg Sodium; 783 mg Potassium; 382 IU Vitamin A; 5 mg ATE Vitamin E; 58 mg Vitamin C; 67 mg Cholesterol

Cantonese Chicken Stir-Fry

This recipe has a very nice light sauce, without the usual soy sauce. It's loaded with vegetables and will fill you up and keep you that way.

2 tablespoons (28 ml) oil

1 cup (122 g) carrot, sliced

2 cups (142 g) broccoli florets

1 cup (160 g) onion, chopped

8 ounces (225 g) mushrooms, sliced

1 cup (70 g) bok choy, chopped

¼ teaspoon ground ginger

¼ teaspoon garlic powder

¼ teaspoon black pepper

3 boneless skinless chicken breast, sliced thinly

1 tablespoon (15 ml) sherry

1 tablespoon (20 g) no-salt-added chili sauce

1 cup (235 ml) low sodium chicken broth

1 tablespoon (8 g) cornstarch

1 cup (195 g) brown rice

In a wok, heat half the oil. Add the carrot, broccoli, onion, and half the spices and stir-fry for 2 minutes. Add the mushrooms and bok choy and stir-fry 1 additional minute. Remove vegetables. Add the remaining oil and heat. Add chicken and remaining spices and stir-fry until chicken is no longer pink. Return the vegetables to the wok. Stir together the sherry, chili sauce, broth, and cornstarch. Add to wok and heat until mixture thickens and begins to bubble. Serve over brown rice cooked according to package directions.

—
4 servings

Each with: 375 Calories (22% from Fat, 22% from Protein, 56% from Carb); 21 g Protein; 9 g Total Fat; 1 g Saturated Fat; 2 g Monounsaturated Fat; 5 g Polyunsaturated Fat; 53 g Carb; 5 g Fiber; 6 g Sugar; 374 mg Phosphorus; 72 mg Calcium; 242 mg Sodium; 797 mg Potassium; 4183 IU Vitamin A; 3 mg ATE Vitamin E; 48 mg Vitamin C; 31 mg Cholesterol

Sure You Can Have Fried Rice

You can have fried rice! The trick is to make the stir-fried rice part of a bigger production that includes lots of meat and vegetables. And that is what this does, starting with low fat, low calorie chicken breasts and then adding lots of vegetables to give you a meal that you can eat.

2 tablespoons (28 ml) olive oil

4 boneless skinless chicken breast, sliced into strips

1 cup (150 g) red bell pepper, chopped

1 cup (124 g) water chestnuts, sliced

2 cups (142 g) broccoli florets

½ cup (50 g) green onion, chopped

3 cups (585 g) cooked brown rice

1 tablespoon (15 ml) rice wine vinegar

¼ cup (60 ml) low sodium soy sauce

1 cup (130 g) frozen peas, thawed

Heat large nonstick skillet over medium heat. Add 1 tablespoon (15 ml) oil. Add chicken, red bell pepper, water chestnuts, broccoli, and green onion. Cook 5 minutes until chicken is cooked through. Remove to a plate. Heat remaining tablespoon (15 ml) of oil in skillet. Add rice and cook 1 minute. Stir in soy sauce, vinegar, and peas; cook 1 minute. Stir in chicken and vegetable mixture.

—
4 servings

Each with: 395 Calories (21% from Fat, 25% from Protein, 54% from Carb); 25 g Protein; 9 g Total Fat; 1 g Saturated Fat; 6 g Monounsaturated Fat; 2 g Polyunsaturated Fat; 54 g Carb; 7 g Fiber; 4 g Sugar; 363 mg Phosphorus; 67 mg Calcium; 725 mg Sodium; 806 mg Potassium; 2637 IU Vitamin A; 4 mg ATE Vitamin E; 112 mg Vitamin C; 41 mg Cholesterol

Sweet and Sour Chicken

This is a simple, quick to prepare version that has a very nice sauce. Because the chicken is stir-fried instead of battered and deep fried, you can actually eat this version and still stay on your diet.

8½ ounces (240 g) pineapple chunks

½ cup (120 g) duck sauce, divided

2 tablespoons (2 g) brown sugar substitute, such as Splenda

¼ cup (60 ml) rice vinegar

1 teaspoon low sodium soy sauce

¼ cup (60 ml) orange juice

1 pound (455 g) boneless skinless chicken breast, cut in ½-inch (1.3 cm) pieces

1 pound (455 g) Asian vegetable mix, frozen

¼ teaspoon ground ginger

1 tablespoon (15 ml) water

2 teaspoons cornstarch

½ cup (80 g) long grain brown rice, cooked according to package directions

Mix juice from pineapple with duck sauce, brown sugar, vinegar, soy sauce, and orange juice. Set aside. In a large skillet with a tight fitting lid, place chicken and sauté until no longer pink on the outside, about 5 minutes. Add ¼ cup (60 ml) of sauce, pineapple chunks, vegetables, and ginger. Cover and simmer until chicken is done and vegetables are crisp-tender. Stir together water and cornstarch. Add to pan with remaining sauce. Cook until mixture is thickened and bubbly. Serve over rice.

—
4 servings

Each with: 387 Calories (5% from Fat, 33% from Protein, 61% from Carb); 32 g Protein; 2 g Total Fat; 1 g Saturated Fat; 1 g Monounsaturated Fat; 1 g Polyunsaturated Fat; 59 g Carb; 6 g Fiber; 9 g Sugar; 322 mg Phosphorus; 64 mg Calcium; 365 mg Sodium; 731 mg Potassium; 4924 IU Vitamin A; 7 mg ATE Vitamin E; 15 mg Vitamin C; 66 mg Cholesterol

Easy Baked Chicken Egg Foo Young

Rather than fried, this egg foo young dish is baked in the oven and saves the fat from the oil. It produces a filling dish full of eggs, chicken, and vegetables at just a little over 300 calories.

CASSEROLE

2 cups (475 ml) egg substitute

1½ cups (150 g) celery, sliced

3 cups (420 g) cooked chicken breast

1½ cups (225 g) red bell pepper, chopped

16 ounces (455 g) bean sprouts, drained

½ cup (64 g) nonfat dry milk powder

2 tablespoons (20 g) onion, chopped

1 tablespoon (4 g) fresh parsley, chopped

⅛ teaspoon black pepper

MUSHROOM SAUCE

2½ tablespoons (20 g) cornstarch

1½ cups (355 ml) low sodium chicken broth, divided

1 tablespoon (15 ml) low sodium soy sauce

4 ounces (115 g) mushrooms, sliced

2 tablespoons (13 g) green onion, sliced

Stir together all casserole ingredients; pour into greased 12 × 8 × 2-inch (30 × 20 × 5 cm) baking dish. Bake at 350°F (180°C, or gas mark 4) for 30 to 35 minutes or until knife inserted in center comes out clean. To make the sauce, combine cornstarch with ¼ cup (60 ml) broth. Heat remaining broth to boiling in a saucepan; gradually whisk in cornstarch, broth mixture, and soy sauce. Cook, stirring until thickened and smooth; add mushrooms and green onion. To serve, cut casserole into squares and top with mushroom sauce.

—
6 servings

Each with: 322 Calories (21% from Fat, 58% from Protein, 22% from Carb); 40 g Protein; 6 g Total Fat; 1 g Unsaturated Fat; 2 g Monounsaturated Fat; 2 g Polyunsaturated Fat; 15 g Carb; 2 g Fiber; 6 g Sugar; 401 mg Phosphorus; 159 mg Calcium; 369 mg Sodium; 980 mg Potassium; 1825 IU Vitamin A; 44 mg ATE Vitamin E; 103 mg Vitamin C; 61 mg Cholesterol

(Just Like at the Mall) Bourbon Chicken

This is a lower sodium, lower fat, lower calorie taste-alike for the kind of chicken they are always giving out samples of at the mall food court. Chicken breasts replace the more common and fattier thighs and sugar substitute sweetens it.

MARINADE

3 tablespoons (45 ml) low sodium soy sauce

½ cup (8 g) brown sugar substitute, such as Splenda

½ teaspoon garlic powder

1 teaspoon ground ginger

2 tablespoons (10 g) dried minced onion

½ cup (120 ml) bourbon

CHICKEN

1 pound (455 g) boneless skinless chicken breast, cut in bite-sized pieces

SIDE DISHES

1½ cups (293 g) brown rice, cooked

1½ cups (107 g) broccoli florets, steamed until crisp-tender

Mix all the marinade ingredients and pour over chicken pieces in a bowl. Cover and refrigerate for several hours or overnight. Bake chicken at 350°F (180°C, or gas mark 4) for one hour in a single layer, basting occasionally. Serve with rice and broccoli.

---

3 servings

Each with: 411 Calories (8% from Fat, 51% from Protein, 41% from Carb); 40 g Protein; 3 g Total Fat; 1 g Unsaturated Fat; 1 g Monounsaturated Fat; 1 g Polyunsaturated Fat; 32 g Carb; 3 g Fiber; 3 g Sugar; 438 mg Phosphorus; 68 mg Calcium; 648 mg Sodium; 688 mg Potassium; 322 IU Vitamin A; 9 mg ATE Vitamin E; 42 mg Vitamin C; 88 mg Cholesterol

TIP:

We like it the way it's shown here, with brown rice and steamed broccoli, but you could substitute other vegetables.

You Can Have (and Love) Chicken Lo Mein

This classic Chinese dish is made more healthy and lower in calories than usual by adding lots more vegetables and using whole wheat pasta. I find that I prefer this to plain white noodles.

8 ounces (225 g) whole wheat spaghetti

4 boneless skinless chicken breasts

6 ounces (170 g) fresh mushrooms, sliced

½ cup (50 g) green onion, sliced

3 tablespoons (42 g) unsalted butter

2 cups (475 ml) low sodium chicken broth

2 teaspoons cornstarch

6 ounces (170 g) snow pea pods

4 ounces (115 g) water chestnuts, sliced

1 pound (455 g) broccoli

2 tablespoons (24 g) pimento, chopped

2 tablespoons (28 ml) low sodium soy sauce

½ teaspoon ground ginger

Prepare spaghetti according to package directions. Drain. In large skillet or Dutch oven, cook chicken, mushrooms, and onion in butter until chicken is tender and liquid is absorbed. Meanwhile, stir together broth and cornstarch. Add to chicken mixture along with cooked spaghetti and remaining ingredients; mix well. Heat through and serve.

—
4 servings

Each with: 353 Calories (27% from Fat, 31% from Protein, 42% from Carb); 29 g Protein; 11 g Total Fat; 6 g Unsaturated Fat; 3 g Monounsaturated Fat; 1 g Polyunsaturated Fat; 39 g Carb; 8 g Fiber; 7 g Sugar; 394 mg Phosphorus; 111 mg Calcium; 398 mg Sodium; 1116 mg Potassium; 1777 IU Vitamin A; 76 mg ATE Vitamin E; 137 mg Vitamin C; 64 mg Cholesterol

Cook All Day, Fill You All Night Chicken Curry

I'm fond of curries. They make a particularly nice slow cooker meal because they fill the house with such a great aroma for you to come home to. This one calls for a number of spices that are typical of curry powder. If you have a favorite curry powder on the shelf, you could substitute a couple of tablespoons (13 g) of that for the other spices.

4 medium potatoes, diced

1 cup (150 g) green bell pepper, coarsely chopped

1 cup (160 g) onion, coarsely chopped

1½ cups (180 g) zucchini, sliced

1½ cups (150 g) cauliflower florets

1 pound (455 g) boneless skinless chicken breast, cubed

2 cups (360 g) no-salt-added tomatoes

1 tablespoon (6 g) coriander

1½ tablespoons (11 g) paprika

1 tablespoon (6 g) ground ginger

¼ teaspoon cayenne pepper

½ teaspoon turmeric

¼ teaspoon cinnamon

⅛ teaspoon ground cloves

1 cup (235 ml) low sodium chicken broth

4 tablespoons (32 g) cornstarch

2 tablespoons (28 ml) cold water

Place vegetables in slow cooker. Place chicken on top. Mix together tomatoes, spices, and chicken broth. Pour over chicken. Cook on low for 8 to 10 hours or on high for 5 to 6 hours. Remove meat and vegetables. Turn heat to high. Stir cornstarch into water. Add to cooker. Cook until sauce is slightly thickened, about 15 to 20 minutes.

—
5 servings

Each with: 406 Calories (6% from Fat, 30% from Protein, 65% from Carb); 30 g Protein; 3 g Total Fat; 1 g Saturated Fat; 0 g Monounsaturated Fat; 1 g Polyunsaturated Fat; 67 g Carb; 9 g Fiber; 10 g Sugar; 434 mg Phosphorus; 95 mg Calcium; 116 mg Sodium; 2121 mg Potassium; 1508 IU Vitamin A; 5 mg ATE Vitamin E; 97 mg Vitamin C; 53 mg Cholesterol

Low Calorie Turkey Meat Loaf Meal

Low fat turkey adds a generous helping of protein to this tasty meat loaf while keeping the calorie count down. Serve with buttermilk mashed potatoes and carrots for a complete meal.

MEAT LOAF

1½ pounds (680 g) ground turkey

1 cup (160 g) onion, chopped

8 ounces (225 g) spinach, thick stems removed and leaves chopped

1 cup (30 g) fresh parsley, chopped

½ cup (60 g) bread crumbs

2 tablespoons (22 g) Dijon mustard

2 tablespoons (28 ml) egg substitute

½ teaspoon black pepper

¼ cup (60 ml) low sodium catsup

POTATOES

2 pounds (900 g) red potatoes, quartered

1 cup (235 ml) low fat buttermilk

1 tablespoon (15 ml) olive oil

3 cups (366 g) carrot, sliced

¼ cup (63 g) low sodium spaghetti sauce

Preheat oven to 400°F (200°C, or gas mark 6). In a bowl, combine the ground turkey, onion, spinach, parsley, bread crumbs, mustard, egg substitute, and black pepper. Transfer the mixture to a baking sheet and form it into a 10-inch (25 cm) loaf. Spread with the ketchup. Bake until cooked through, 45 to 50 minutes. Meanwhile, place the potatoes in a large pot of enough water to cover and bring to a boil. Reduce heat and simmer until tender, 15 to 18 minutes. Drain the potatoes and return them to the pot. Mash with the low fat buttermilk, oil, and ¼ teaspoon black pepper. Cook carrots in boiling water until tender. Serve the meat loaf with the potatoes and carrots and pass the spaghetti sauce.

—

6 servings

Each with: 385 Calories (14% from Fat, 37% from Protein, 49% from Carb); 36 g Protein; 6 g Total Fat; 1 g Unsaturated Fat; 2 g Monounsaturated Fat; 1 g Polyunsaturated Fat; 48 g Carb; 7 g Fiber; 11 g Sugar; 448 mg Phosphorus; 183 mg Calcium; 386 mg Sodium; 1738 mg Potassium; 12 284 IU Vitamin A; 3 mg ATE Vitamin E; 62 mg Vitamin C; 70 mg Cholesterol

Turkey and Barley Stuffed Green Peppers

Stuffed peppers can turn out to be diet nightmare. Here we've avoided that by using turkey instead of beef and limiting the cheese and making it low fat. But the flavor is still rich and the added volume of the mushrooms and onions will help to fill you up.

1 tablespoon (15 ml) olive oil

1 pound (455 g) ground turkey

2 cups (140 g) mushrooms, chopped

1 cup (160 g) onion, chopped

1 cup (157 g) cooked pearl barley

2 tablespoons (8 g) fresh parsley, chopped

¼ teaspoon dried thyme

¼ teaspoon black pepper

½ cup (58 g) low fat Monterey Jack cheese, shredded

4 green bell peppers

1 cup (245 g) no-salt-added tomato sauce

Preheat oven to 350°F (180°C, or gas mark 4) degrees. Heat the oil in a large skillet. Add turkey, mushrooms, and onion and cook, stirring until the onions are browned and turkey is no longer pink. Stir in the barley, parsley, thyme, and black pepper. Stir in the cheese; set aside. Cut off the tops of the peppers; remove and discard the seeds. Spoon ¼ of the mixture into each pepper. Stand the peppers upright in a baking dish just large enough to accommodate them. Pour the sauce over the peppers. Bake 30 minutes or until the peppers are tender.

—
4 servings

Each with: 400 Calories (17% from Fat, 39% from Protein, 44% from Carb); 39 g Protein; 8 g Total Fat; 2 g Saturated Fat; 3 g Monounsaturated Fat; 1 g Polyunsaturated Fat; 44 g Carb; 10 g Fiber; 5 g Sugar; 494 mg Phosphorus; 120 mg Calcium; 188 mg Sodium; 971 mg Potassium; 417 IU Vitamin A; 10 mg ATE Vitamin E; 14 mg Vitamin C; 72 mg Cholesterol

Dinners: Beef

Unlike the chicken and turkey of the previous chapter, beef has a reputation of being bad for you. It tends to be high in saturated fat and that is doubly bad, because it not only adds calories, but it is a contributor to heart problems. However, this doesn't have to be the case if you are careful about the cuts of beef you use. Many of the recipes in this chapter call for low fat cuts of beef like round steak. If they are cooked properly, they can be just as good as the fatter cuts (which also are usually more expensive, so that's another advantage). The recipes using ground beef call for extra lean. I usually buy either the 93% lean or for an even leaner and cheaper alternative buy cuts like top round steak, often called London broil, and grind it myself. We do still try to limit the number of meals we have with beef, but it has a place in our meal plan.

Sirloin Steak with Golden Fried Zucchini

Do you think that you can't have good steak while trying to lose weight? Think again. The trick to being able to eat steak like this sirloin is to limit the portion size and team it with other healthy filling foods like the zucchini and whole wheat couscous featured here.

2 tablespoons (28 ml) olive oil

1½ pound (680 g) sirloin steak

½ teaspoon black pepper

6 small zucchini,
halved lengthwise

1 teaspoon lemon zest, grated

½ teaspoon garlic, finely
chopped

3 tablespoons (20 g) fresh herbs,
such as parsley, cilantro, or basil

2 tablespoons (14 g)
bread crumbs

12 ounces (340 g) whole
wheat couscous

Heat 1 tablespoon (15 ml) of the oil in a large skillet over medium-high heat. Season the steak with black pepper. Cook the steak to desired doneness, 4 to 5 minutes per side for medium-rare. Transfer to a cutting board. Let rest 10 minutes before slicing. Meanwhile, return the pan to medium heat and add 2 teaspoons of the oil. Cook the zucchini, cut-side down, covered, until browned and tender, about 6 minutes. Cut crosswise into ½-inch (1.3 cm) pieces and divide among plates. In a bowl, combine the lemon zest, garlic, herbs, bread crumbs, and remaining oil. Sprinkle the mixture over the zucchini. Serve the zucchini and couscous with the steak.

—
6 servings

Each with: 413 Calories (55% from Fat, 26% from Protein, 19% from Carb); 27 g Protein; 25 g Total Fat; 9 g Unsaturated Fat; 12 g Monounsaturated Fat; 1 g Polyunsaturated Fat; 19 g Carb; 3 g Fiber; 2 g Sugar; 266 mg Phosphorus; 62 mg Calcium; 89 mg Sodium; 717 mg Potassium; 306 IU Vitamin A; 0 mg ATE Vitamin E; 24 mg Vitamin C; 74 mg Cholesterol

Wine Sauced Steak

Kind of like a combination of beef Burgundy and Swiss steak, this dish is sure to please. And it's also low in calories while providing a filling meal.

2 pound (900 g) beef round steak

2 tablespoons (16 g) all purpose flour

½ teaspoon black pepper

2 tablespoons (28 ml) olive oil

1 cup (160 g) onion, chopped

½ cup (61 g) carrot, sliced

14 ounces (390 g) no-salt-added tomatoes

¾ cup (175 ml) dry red wine

½ teaspoon garlic, minced

¼ cup (60 ml) water

2 tablespoons (16 g) all purpose flour

3 cups (585 g) brown rice, cooked

Trim fat from steak; cut meat into 6 equal pieces. Coat with mixture of flour and black pepper. Pound steak to ½-inch (1.3 cm) thickness using a meat mallet. Brown meat in hot oil; drain. Place onion and carrot in slow cooker. Place meat atop. Combine undrained tomatoes, wine, and garlic. Pour over meat. Cover; cook on low heat setting for 8 to 10 hours. Transfer meat and vegetables to serving platter. Reserve 1½ cups (355 ml) of the cooking liquid for wine sauce. To make the wine sauce, pour reserved liquid into saucepan. Blend cold water slowly into flour; stir into liquid. Cook and stir until thickened and bubbly. Serve meat and vegetables over rice. Spoon some sauce over meat; pass remaining sauce.

—

6 servings

Each with: 410 Calories (25% from Fat, 40% from Protein, 36% from Carb); 38 g Protein; 10 g Total Fat; 3 g Unsaturated Fat; 6 g Monounsaturated Fat; 1 g Polyunsaturated Fat; 34 g Carb; 3 g Fiber; 4 g Sugar; 440 mg Phosphorus; 48 mg Calcium; 96 mg Sodium; 921 mg Potassium; 1372 IU Vitamin A; 0 mg ATE Vitamin E; 12 mg Vitamin C; 86 mg Cholesterol

Pure Comfort Beef and Barley Casserole

This quick casserole has a great flavor from a unique combination of ingredients. Use of extra lean ground beef helps to hold down the calories, while whole grain barley and vegetables pack in the nutrition.

⅓ cup (67 g) pearl barley

1 pound (455 g) extra lean ground beef, browned

1 cup (160 g) onion, cut up

1 cup (122 g) carrot, sliced

2 tablespoons (40 g) molasses

2 tablespoons (28 ml) low sodium soy sauce

In a 2-quart (1.9 L) casserole, mix barley, browned beef, onion, carrot, and molasses. Mix well. Add enough water to cover. Bake at 350°F (180°C, or gas mark 4) for 1 hour covered. Before serving, stir in soy sauce. Mix. You may have to add more water during baking.

—
4 servings

Each with: 384 Calories (47% from Fat, 25% from Protein, 28% from Carb); 24 g Protein; 20 g Total Fat; 8 g Unsaturated Fat; 8 g Monounsaturated Fat; 1 g Polyunsaturated Fat; 27 g Carb; 4 g Fiber; 9 g Sugar; 234 mg Phosphorus; 55 mg Calcium; 369 mg Sodium; 720 mg Potassium; 3856 IU Vitamin A; 0 mg ATE Vitamin E; 4 mg Vitamin C; 78 mg Cholesterol

Squash That Hamburger

OK, maybe I've been at this too long tonight, but Hamburger Zucchini Casserole sounded so mundane. And this tastes anything but mundane. It a warm, filling tasty treat full of good things like extra lean ground beef, squash, and cheese. So squash your resistance and give it a try.

6 cups (720 g) zucchini, diced

1 pound (455 g) extra lean ground beef

1 cup (160 g) onion, chopped

2 cups (390 g) brown rice, cooked

1 teaspoon dried oregano

1 teaspoon garlic powder

16 ounces (455 g) fat-free cottage cheese

1 can (10¾ ounces, or 305 g) low sodium cream of mushroom soup

1 cup (115 g) low fat Monterey Jack cheese, shredded

Cook squash and drain well. Sauté beef and onion. Add rice and seasoning to beef. Place half of squash in 2½-quart (2.4 L) casserole. Cover with beef mix and spoon over the cottage cheese. Add squash and spread on soup. Sprinkle with cheese. Bake at 350°F (180°C, or gas mark 4) for 35 to 45 minutes, uncovered.

—
4 servings

Each with: 445 Calories (42% from Fat, 27% from Protein, 31% from Carb); 35 g Protein; 24 g Total Fat; 10 g Unsaturated Fat; 10 g Monounsaturated Fat; 2 g Polyunsaturated Fat; 40 g Carb; 5 g Fiber; 7 g Sugar; 516 mg Phosphorus; 205 mg Calcium; 569 mg Sodium; 1243 mg Potassium; 464 IU Vitamin A; 21 mg ATE Vitamin E; 34 mg Vitamin C; 87 mg Cholesterol

Stuffed Red Peppers

Red peppers contain a lot more vitamin A than green ones, so why not use them for stuffed peppers. I like the flavor better too.

6 red bell peppers

½ cup (60 g) bread crumbs

1 cup (235 ml) nonfat evaporated milk

¾ cup (120 g) chopped onion

2 tablespoons (28 ml) olive oil

1½ pounds (680 g) extra lean ground beef

¼ cup (25 g) scallions

2 cups (475 g) water

Blanch red bell peppers, cut off tops, and finely chop as much of the tops as possible. Combine bread crumbs and evaporated milk and let soak. Cook onion in oil until tender. Combine all ingredients and stuff peppers. Place in a dish, add water, and cook at 375°F (190°C, or gas mark 5) for one hour.

—

6 servings

Each with: 377 Calories (58% from Fat, 27% from Protein, 14% from Carb); 26 g Protein; 24 g Total Fat; 8 g Saturated Fat; 12 g Monounsaturated Fat; 1 g Polyunsaturated Fat; 14 g Carb; 2 g Fiber; 9 g Sugar; 273 mg Phosphorus; 152 mg Calcium; 154 mg Sodium; 665 mg Potassium; 2543 IU Vitamin A; 51 mg ATE Vitamin E; 144 mg Vitamin C; 80 mg Cholesterol

Better for You Beef Stroganoff

In this recipe, we've limited the amount of beef (but only to what a serving is supposed to be) and added the nontraditional carrots for a nutritional boost. This makes a great comfort food meal for a chilly evening.

1¼ pound (570 g) beef round steak

2 tablespoons (28 ml) olive oil

1½ cups (105 g) mushrooms, sliced

1 cup (110 g) carrot, shredded

½ teaspoon sherry flavoring

¾ cup (125 ml) low sodium beef broth

½ cup (115 g) fat-free sour cream

3 cups (480 g) egg noodles

Cut meat into ¼-inch (6 mm) strips. Heat oil in skillet. Brown meat quickly, 2 to 4 minutes. Remove meat. Add mushrooms and carrot to skillet. Cook for 2 to 3 minutes. Remove mushrooms. Add sherry and broth to skillet and cook until liquid is reduced to about ⅓ cup (80 ml). Stir in sour cream. Stir in meat and mushrooms. Heat through without boiling.

—

6 servings

Each with: 376 Calories (32% from Fat, 43% from Protein, 25% from Carb); 40 g Protein; 13 g Total Fat; 4 g Unsaturated Fat; 6 g Monounsaturated Fat; 1 g Polyunsaturated Fat; 23 g Carb; 2 g Fiber; 2 g Sugar; 314 mg Phosphorus; 44 mg Calcium; 89 mg Sodium; 504 mg Potassium; 2660 IU Vitamin A; 25 mg ATE Vitamin E; 2 mg Vitamin C; 119 mg Cholesterol

Beef Stew Hungarian Style

Similar to what is usually called beef paprikash, this stew has just the right amount of spice to satisfy and just few enough calories to be perfect for our plans.

2 tablespoons (28 ml) olive oil

1 cup (160 g) onion, chopped

1½ pound (680 g) beef round steak, cubed

½ teaspoon black pepper, coarsely ground

1 tablespoon (7 g) paprika

½ teaspoon dried marjoram, crumbled

½ teaspoon caraway seeds

1 cup (122 g) carrot, cut in 2-inch (5 cm) pieces

½ cup (50 g) celery, cut in 2-inch (5 cm) pieces

1 cup (150 g) green bell pepper, cut in 1-inch (2.5 cm) pieces

1 cup (160 g) tomatoes, cut up

8 ounces (225 g) mushrooms, sliced

¾ cup (180 g) fat-free sour cream

Heat oil and sauté onion until soft and golden. Add beef, stir, and then add all the other ingredients except for sour cream. Cover, reduce heat, and simmer until tender, up to 2 hours. Stir occasionally and add water if needed. Serve with a dollop of sour cream.

—
4 servings

Each with: 394 Calories (42% from Fat, 43% from Protein, 14% from Carb); 42 g Protein; 19 g Total Fat; 6 g Unsaturated Fat; 9 g Monounsaturated Fat; 1 g Polyunsaturated Fat; 14 g Carb; 4 g Fiber; 5 g Sugar; 474 mg Phosphorus; 123 mg Calcium; 168 mg Sodium; 1089 mg Potassium; 5376 IU Vitamin A; 45 mg ATE Vitamin E; 46 mg Vitamin C; 96 mg Cholesterol

TIP:

If you can find it, use Hungarian sweet paprika.

Pot Roast New Orleans Style

A taste of old New Orleans, this beef is nicely spiced and cooked with the traditional onion, celery and green bell pepper. Those Cajuns must know something about healthy cooking.

6 cups (1.2 kg) brown rice, cooked

2½ pound (1.1 kg) beef round roast

¼ teaspoon cayenne pepper

½ teaspoon black pepper

2 teaspoons olive oil

1 cup (160 g) onion, chopped

1 cup (100 g) celery, chopped

1 cup (150 g) green bell pepper, chopped

2 tablespoons (16 g) all p urpose flour

1 teaspoon garlic, minced

28 ounces (785 g) no-salt-added tomatoes

1 cup (235 ml) low sodium beef broth

½ teaspoon dried thyme

½ teaspoon basil

1 bay leaf

Prepare rice according to package directions. Rub meat all over with cayenne pepper and black pepper. In Dutch oven, heat oil and brown meat. Take out meat and sauté vegetables. Add flour to vegetables and cook 2 minutes, stirring constantly. Add garlic, tomatoes, broth, thyme, basil, and bay leaf. Stir until well blended. Place meat back in Dutch oven. Bring liquid to boil on high heat. Reduce heat to simmer, cover, and cook 2½ to 3 hours. Remove bay leaf. Slice meat and serve sauce and vegetables over both meat and rice.

—
8 servings

Each with: 399 Calories (18% from Fat, 37% from Protein, 45% from Carb); 37 g Protein; 8 g Total Fat; 2 g Unsaturated Fat; 4 g Monounsaturated Fat; 1 g Polyunsaturated Fat; 44 g Carb; 5 g Fiber; 4 g Sugar; 459 mg Phosphorus; 93 mg Calcium; 130 mg Sodium; 980 mg Potassium; 302 IU Vitamin A; 0 mg ATE Vitamin E; 31 mg Vitamin C; 71 mg Cholesterol

TIP:

Feel free to add more cayenne pepper if you like things spicier (or more like real Cajun food).

Mostly Eggplant Stew

This recipe is a nice variation on the beef stew theme, with different vegetables and spices. The combination is part Mediterranean, but the cumin adds a bit of a Latin taste. The generous amount of vegetables just soaks up the flavor, making this a family favorite around our house.

2 pound (900 g) beef round steak, cubed

2 tablespoons (28 ml) olive oil

2 cups (360 g) no-salt-added tomatoes

1 cup (160 g) onion, chopped

2 tablespoons (32 g) no-salt-added tomato paste

½ teaspoon dried oregano

½ teaspoon dried basil

½ teaspoon ground cumin

¼ teaspoon red pepper

½ teaspoon garlic powder

1 cup (235 ml) water

1 medium potato, peeled and cubed

1 cup (235 ml) white wine

2 eggplants, peeled and cubed

2 cups (240 g) zucchini, sliced

8 ounces (225 g) mushrooms, sliced

In a Dutch oven, brown half the beef at a time in the oil. Drain and return all meat to the pan. Add tomatoes, onion, tomato paste, and spices. Stir in water. Bring to a boil. Reduce heat and simmer, covered, for 45 minutes. Add potato and wine. Cover and simmer 10 minutes more. Stir in eggplant, zucchini, and mushrooms. Cover and simmer until meat and vegetables are tender, 15 to 20 minutes.

—
6 servings

Each with: 386 Calories (25% from Fat, 43% from Protein, 32% from Carb); 40 g Protein; 10 g Total Fat; 2 g Saturated Fat; 5 g Monounsaturated Fat; 1 g Polyunsaturated Fat; 29 g Carb; 9 g Fiber; 10 g Sugar; 472 mg Phosphorus; 70 mg Calcium; 107 mg Sodium; 1637 mg Potassium; 331 IU Vitamin A; 0 mg ATE Vitamin E; 30 mg Vitamin C; 86 mg Cholesterol

Healthy, Hearty Roast Beef Hash

This could also be eaten for breakfast, but it's loaded with lots of vegetables and makes an easy dinner. You can use whatever leftover roast beef you have, trimmed of fat. We've also made it using part of a leftover smoked beef roast.

1 pound (455 g) roast beef, cooked and chopped

1 medium potato, peeled and diced

1 cup (160 g) onion, chopped

1 cup (150 g) green bell pepper, chopped

¼ cup (25 g) celery, chopped

1 tablespoon (9 g) dry mustard

1 tablespoon (9 g) garlic powder

¼ tablespoon dried thyme

¾ cup (175 ml) low sodium beef broth

Combine all ingredients and pack into a well greased baking pan. Cover with foil and bake at 375°F (190°C, or gas mark 5) for 45 minutes. Uncover, turn oven to broil, and brown the top.

—

3 servings

Each with: 439 Calories (31% from Fat, 41% from Protein, 28% from Carb); 45 g Protein; 15 g Total Fat; 5 g Unsaturated Fat; 6 g Monounsaturated Fat; 1 g Polyunsaturated Fat; 30 g Carb; 4 g Fiber; 5 g Sugar; 332 mg Phosphorus; 52 mg Calcium; 105 mg Sodium; 917 mg Potassium; 246 IU Vitamin A; 0 mg ATE Vitamin E; 52 mg Vitamin C; 159 mg Cholesterol

Oven Smoked Roast

Spices and liquid smoke give this roast its right-out-of-the-smoker flavor.

2½ pound (1.1 kg) beef round roast

2 cups (475 ml) low sodium beef broth

¼ cup (60 ml) low sodium soy sauce

¼ cup (60 ml) lemon juice

1 tablespoon (10 g) garlic, minced

1 tablespoon (15 ml) Liquid Smoke

8 ounces (225 g) egg noodles, cooked

6 cups (600 g) green beans, cooked

Place roast in roasting pan. Combine broth, soy sauce, lemon juice, garlic, and Liquid Smoke in bowl. Mix well. Pour over roast. Marinate in refrigerator overnight. Bake covered at 300°F (150°C, or gas mark 3) for 2½ hours. Bake uncovered for 30 minutes longer. Serve with noodles and green beans.

—

8 servings

Each with: 327 Calories (18% from Fat, 47% from Protein, 34% from Carb); 38 g Protein; 7 g Total Fat; 2 g Unsaturated Fat; 3 g Monounsaturated Fat; 1 g Polyunsaturated Fat; 28 g Carb; 4 g Fiber; 2 g Sugar; 418 mg Phosphorus; 76 mg Calcium; 400 mg Sodium; 811 mg Potassium; 588 IU Vitamin A; 5 mg ATE Vitamin E; 17 mg Vitamin C; 98 mg Cholesterol

One Dish Lasagna Pie

This recipe is a variation of the Bisquick impossible pies that make their own crust as they bake. In this case, we've increased the vegetables and held down the fat to give you a meal that is filling, tasty, and nutritious.

1 pound (455 g) extra lean ground beef

1 cup (245 g) low sodium spaghetti sauce

⅓ cup (85 g) ricotta cheese

3 tablespoons (15 g) Parmesan cheese, grated

1 tablespoon (15 ml) skim milk

1 cup (120 g) zucchini, sliced

1 cup (150 g) red bell pepper, sliced

1 cup (160 g) onion, sliced

1 cup (150 g) fresh mozzarella, grated

½ cup (63 g) all purpose flour

¾ teaspoon baking powder

2 tablespoons (28 g) unsalted butter

1 cup (235 ml) skim milk

½ cup (120 ml) egg substitute

Preheat oven to 400°F (200°C, or gas mark 6). Grease a 9-inch (23 cm) pie plate. Cook beef in a 10-inch (25 cm) skillet over medium heat, stirring occasionally, until brown; drain. Stir in ½ cup (123 g) spaghetti sauce; heat until bubbly. Stir together ricotta cheese, Parmesan cheese, and 1 tablespoon (15 ml) skim milk. Spread half of the beef mixture in pie plate. Drop cheese mixture by spoonfuls onto the beef mixture. Top with vegetables. Sprinkle with ½ cup (75 g) of the mozzarella cheese. Top with remaining beef mixture. Stir together flour and baking powder. Cut in butter. Stir in skim milk and egg substitute until blended. Pour into pie plate. Bake 30 to 35 minutes or until knife inserted in center comes out clean. Sprinkle with remaining ½ cup (75 g) mozzarella cheese. Bake 2 to 3 minutes longer or until cheese is melted.

—
4 servings

Each with: 369 Calories (41% from Fat, 25% from Protein, 34% from Carb); 23 g Protein; 17 g Total Fat; 10 g Saturated Fat; 5 g Monounsaturated Fat; 2 g Polyunsaturated Fat; 32 g Carb; 3 g Fiber; 5 g Sugar; 494 mg Phosphorus; 535 mg Calcium; 485 mg Sodium; 855 mg Potassium; 2172 IU Vitamin A; 160 mg ATE Vitamin E; 85 mg Vitamin C; 45 mg Cholesterol

Southwestern Beef with Chili Dumplings

Here's a great southwestern meal in a pot. With the dumplings, nothing else is even needed. Well-trimmed round steak helps to hold down the fat and calories while beans give a nutrition boost.

1½ pounds (680 g) beef round steak

¼ cup (31 g) all purpose flour

1 teaspoon chili powder

½ teaspoon ground cumin

¼ teaspoon black pepper

2 tablespoons (28 ml) olive oil

1 cup (160 g) onion, chopped

2 cups (512 g) kidney beans, cooked

10 ounces (280 g) frozen corn

Dumplings

2 cups (250 g) all purpose flour

1 teaspoon chili powder

1 tablespoon (14 g) baking powder

3 tablespoons (42 g) unsalted butter

¾ cup (175 ml) skim milk

Trim fat from beef and cut into 1-inch (2.5 cm) cubes. Shake meat with flour, chili powder, cumin, and black pepper in a zipper baggie to coat well. Heat oil in a large Dutch oven. Add beef cubes to oil, a few at a time, and brown. Stir in onion and sauté until soft. Return beef to pot. Drain liquid from beans into a large measuring container and add water to make 3 cups (700 ml). Stir into beef mixture and cover. Heat to boiling. Lower heat and simmer for 2 hours or until beef is tender. Stir in corn and beans; heat to boiling again. In large bowl, combine flour, chili powder, and baking powder. Cut in butter until mixture resembles coarse crumbs. Add skim milk all at once and stir with a fork until evenly moist. Drop batter by tablespoon on top of boiling stew. Cook uncovered, 10 minutes. Cover. Cook 10 minutes longer or until dumplings are done.

—

8 servings

Each with: 412 Calories (25% from Fat, 29% from Protein, 46% from Carb); 30 g Protein; 12 g Total Fat; 4 g Unsaturated Fat; 5 g Monounsaturated Fat; 1 g Polyunsaturated Fat; 48 g Carb; 7 g Fiber; 2 g Sugar; 394 mg Phosphorus; 197 mg Calcium; 267 mg Sodium; 723 mg Potassium; 442 IU Vitamin A; 50 mg ATE Vitamin E; 5 mg Vitamin C; 51 mg Cholesterol

Mexican Stacks

Tasty tortillas layered with an extra lean beef mixture give you the flavor of Mexico without the calories. And that should make lots of people happy.

1 pound (455 g) extra lean ground beef

1 package taco seasoning

5 whole wheat tortillas, 6-inch (15 cm)

5 ounces (140 g) low fat cheddar cheese, grated

5 ounces (140 g) low fat Monterey Jack cheese, grated

4 ounces (115 g) olives, sliced

4 ounces (115 g) green chilies, chopped

½ cup (80 g) onion, chopped

1 teaspoon olive oil

Preheat oven to 350°F (180°C, or gas mark 4). Brown meat. Add taco seasoning according to directions on package. Layer tortillas in 9-inch (23 cm) pie pan sprayed with nonstick vegetable oil spray. Begin with tortillas. Spread with ¼ of meat, cheeses, olives, chilies, and onion. Repeat 4 times. Brush top tortilla with olive oil. Bake for 30 minutes or until top is golden brown.

6 servings

Each with: 420 Calories (47% from Fat, 28% from Protein, 25% from Carb); 29 g Protein; 22 g Total Fat; 8 g Unsaturated Fat; 10 g Monounsaturated Fat; 1 g Polyunsaturated Fat; 25 g Carb; 2 g Fiber; 1 g Sugar; 389 mg Phosphorus; 275 mg Calcium; 761 mg Sodium; 338 mg Potassium; 198 IU Vitamin A; 28 mg ATE Vitamin E; 7 mg Vitamin C; 62 mg Cholesterol

Fajita Tacos

The filling says fajita, but the corn tortilla says taco. In reality, it doesn't matter because there is way too much filling to stick in two tortillas anyway, so you'll probably end up eating it with a fork.

2 tablespoons (28 ml) olive oil

2 teaspoons ground cumin

1 teaspoon garlic, minced

1 pound (455 g) beef round steak, cut in strips

1½ cups (225 g) green bell pepper

1½ cups (225 g) red bell pepper

1 cup (160 g) onion, sliced

8 corn tortillas

½ cup (130 g) salsa

¼ cup (60 g) fat-free sour cream

In a skillet, sauté olive oil, cumin, and garlic for 1 minute. Add steak strips and cook about 5 minutes. Add green and red bell pepper and onion slices and cook for another 8 minutes. Place mixture in tortillas and fold. Top with salsa and sour cream.

4 servings

Each with: 365 Calories (34% from Fat, 33% from Protein, 33% from Carb); 31 g Protein; 14 g Total Fat; 4 g Unsaturated Fat; 8 g Monounsaturated Fat; 2 g Polyunsaturated Fat; 31 g Carb; 5 g Fiber; 7 g Sugar; 436 mg Phosphorus; 144 mg Calcium; 285 mg Sodium; 863 mg Potassium; 2244 IU Vitamin A; 15 mg ATE Vitamin E; 159 mg Vitamin C; 58 mg Cholesterol

Easy Slow Cooker Enchiladas Casserole

This is an easy to fix enchilada-style casserole that cooks in the slow cooker and leaves you with a house full of delicious aromas. Beans and vegetables kick up the nutrition and the taste of the Mexican-influenced treat.

1 pound (455 g) extra lean ground beef

1 cup (160 g) onion, chopped

1½ cups (225 g) red bell pepper, chopped

1½ cups (225 g) green bell pepper, chopped

10 ounces (280 g) frozen corn

2 cups (342 g) pinto beans

2 cups (344 g) black beans

2 cups (360 g) no-salt-added tomatoes

4 ounces (115 g) diced green chilies

1 teaspoon chili powder

1 teaspoon ground cumin

½ teaspoon black pepper

3 ounces (85 g) low fat cheddar cheese, shredded

3 ounces (85 g) low fat Monterey Jack cheese, shredded

6 whole wheat tortillas, 6-inch (15 cm)

In a nonstick skillet, brown beef, onion, and green and red bell peppers. Add remaining ingredients except cheese and tortillas, Bring to a boil. Reduce heat. Cover and simmer for 10 minutes. Combine cheeses in a bowl. In slow cooker, layer about ¾ cup beef mixture, one tortilla, and about ¼ cup (29 g) cheese. Repeat layers until all ingredients are used. Cover. Cook on low for 5 to 7 hours.

—
8 servings

Each with: 406 Calories (32% from Fat, 24% from Protein, 44% from Carb); 25 g Protein; 15 g Total Fat; 6 g Saturated Fat; 6 g Monounsaturated Fat; 1 g Polyunsaturated Fat; 45 g Carb; 8 g Fiber; 6 g Sugar; 351 mg Phosphorus; 183 mg Calcium; 405 mg Sodium; 769 mg Potassium; 1291 IU Vitamin A; 13 mg ATE Vitamin E; 93 mg Vitamin C; 44 mg Cholesterol

Mexican Steak Salad

If you have leftover London broil or other beef, this salad is a great tasting, healthy way to use it. So you really should plan to have some leftover beef. The Mexican taste is a real pleaser, and the nutrition will make everyone happy.

½ cup (115 g) sour cream

½ cup (130 g) salsa

2 tablespoons (2 g) cilantro, divided

1 cup (256 g) kidney beans, rinsed and drained

½ cup (56 g) low fat Monterey Jack cheese

¼ cup (25 g) green onion, sliced

8 ounces (225 g) beef round steak, cooked and sliced

1 small head iceberg lettuce, shredded

5 radishes, thinly sliced

1 avocado, peeled and sliced

2 ounces (28 g) tortilla chips

In a small bowl, combine sour cream, salsa, and 1 tablespoon (1 g) cilantro; set aside. In a medium bowl, combine beans, cheese, green onion, and remaining 1 tablespoon (1 g) cilantro. To serve, arrange bean mixture, beef, lettuce, radishes, avocado, and tortilla chips on four individual plates. Serve topped with the sour cream and salsa mixture.

—
4 servings

Each with: 368 Calories (38% from Fat, 27% from Protein, 35% from Carb); 26 g Protein; 16 g Total Fat; 5 g Saturated Fat; 7 g Monounsaturated Fat; 2 g Polyunsaturated Fat; 33 g Carb; 9 g Fiber; 6 g Sugar; 418 mg Phosphorus; 201 mg Calcium; 453 mg Sodium; 1111 mg Potassium; 1198 IU Vitamin A; 40 mg ATE Vitamin E; 20 mg Vitamin C; 48 mg Cholesterol

Easy to Fix, Easy on Your Diet Beef Burgundy

This is a great beef and noodles dish. It's easy to prepare in your slow cooker. And it's easy on your diet because the long slow cooking lets you use a cheaper, leaner cut of beef and still end up with a tender, delicious meal. This meal is a perfect example of how you can eat a lot of food that seems to be rich but is still low in calories.

4 slices low sodium bacon

2 pound (900 g) beef round steak, cut in 1-inch (2.5 cm) cubes

2 cups (244 g) carrot, cut into chunks

2 cups (320 g) onion, sliced

½ cup (63 g) all-purpose flour

½ teaspoon marjoram

¼ teaspoon garlic powder

¼ teaspoon black pepper

1½ cups (355 ml) low sodium beef broth

½ cup (120 ml) burgundy wine

1 tablespoon (15 ml) Worcestershire sauce

12 ounces (340 g) mushrooms, sliced

16 ounces (455 g) egg noodles, uncooked

2 tablespoons (8 g) fresh parsley

6 cups (600 g) green beans

Cook bacon until crisp; drain and crumble. Place beef, bacon, carrot, and onion in the bottom of the slow cooker. Whisk together flour, marjoram, garlic, and black pepper with broth, wine, and Worcestershire sauce. Pour mixture into cooker. Cook on high for 1 hour. Reduce to low and cook for 5 to 6 hours. Add mushrooms. Cook on high for 30 minutes or until mushrooms are tender. While mushrooms are cooking, prepare noodles and beans according to package directions. Serve beef over noodles with beans on the side.

—

8 servings

Each with: 352 Calories (17% from Fat, 41% from Protein, 41% from Carb); 36 g Protein; 7 g Total Fat; 2 g Unsaturated Fat; 2 g Monounsaturated Fat; 1 g Polyunsaturated Fat; 35 g Carb; 5 g Fiber; 5 g Sugar; 420 mg Phosphorus; 87 mg Calcium; 245 mg Sodium; 997 mg Potassium; 4518 IU Vitamin A; 4 mg ATE Vitamin E; 24 mg Vitamin C; 75 mg Cholesterol

Grilled Soy and Ginger Flank Steak with Vegetables

This is a sort of Asian flavored meal, with the soy sauce and ginger. But the ingredients, steak and corn on the cob, are classic American. But the important part is that it works, giving you a meal that is both healthy and flavorful.

1 pound (455 g) flank steak

1 tablespoon (6 g) fresh ginger, minced

2 teaspoons garlic, minced

¼ cup (60 ml) low sodium soy sauce

3 tablespoons (45 ml) dry red wine

1 tablespoon (20 g) honey

4 ears corn

4 red bell peppers, halved

8 ounces (225 g) mushrooms, whole

Rinse the meat and pat dry. Place steak in a 1 gallon (3.8 L) plastic freezer bag and add the remaining ingredients except the vegetables. Seal bag and turn to coat. Lightly oil a barbecue grill and preheat to very hot. Remove the steak from the bag, reserving marinade for vegetables. Cook steak, turning once, until done as you like it, about 15 minutes total for medium-rare. To serve, slice diagonally across the grain into thin slices. Add husked corn, halved and seeded red bell peppers, and mushrooms to the marinade after removing the steak and then cook on the grill, turning occasionally until slightly browned.

—

4 servings

Each with: 418 Calories (24% from Fat, 36% from Protein, 40% from Carb); 39 g Protein; 12 g Total Fat; 4 g Saturated Fat; 4 g Monounsaturated Fat; 1 g Polyunsaturated Fat; 43 g Carb; 7 g Fiber; 16 g Sugar; 427 mg Phosphorus; 37 mg Calcium; 620 mg Sodium; 1140 mg Potassium; 4667 IU Vitamin A; 0 mg ATE Vitamin E; 293 mg Vitamin C; 62 mg Cholesterol

Beef and Tomato Curry (Plus Other Good Stuff)

Beef, tomatoes, and other vegetables are simmered in a mild curry sauce to make this tasty dish. Like many soups and stews, it offers great nutrition and volume for the calories. Brown rice adds extra nutrition and filling power.

1 pound (455 g) beef round steak

½ cup (120 ml) low sodium beef broth

1½ cups (270 g) tomatoes, coarsely chopped

1 cup (150 g) green bell pepper, cut in 1-inch (2.5 cm) pieces

8 ounces (225 g) mushrooms, sliced

1½ cups (240 g) onion, coarsely chopped

1½ cups (180 g) zucchini, sliced

1 teaspoon curry powder

1 tablespoon (8 g) cornstarch

1 tablespoon (15 ml) water

1 cup (195 g) brown rice, cooked according to package directions

Cut meat into 1 × 2-inch (2.5 × 5 cm) strips. Spray skillet with nonstick vegetable oil spray. Cook meat in broth until tender. Add tomatoes, peeled and cut up, green bell pepper, onion, mushrooms, zucchini, and curry powder and heat to boiling. Cover and cook on medium for 3 to 5 minutes. Mix cornstarch and water. Stir into mixture and cook until thick and boiling. Serve over hot cooked rice.

—

4 servings

Each with: 391 Calories (13% from Fat, 34% from Protein, 53% from Carb); 34 g Protein; 6 g Total Fat; 2 g Saturated Fat; 2 g Monounsaturated Fat; 1 g Polyunsaturated Fat; 52 g Carb; 5 g Fiber; 6 g Sugar; 511 mg Phosphorus; 47 mg Calcium; 95 mg Sodium; 1137 mg Potassium; 585 IU Vitamin A; 0 mg ATE Vitamin E; 58 mg Vitamin C; 65 mg Cholesterol

Not Your Irish Corned Beef and Cabbage

Unlike the traditional version, this corned beef and cabbage cooks in a spicy tomato sauce. But don't let that stop you. It tastes good, is full of nutrition, and is very low in calories.

1 large cabbage, sliced in ½-inch (1.3 cm) slices

½ cup (120 ml) water

1 cup (160 g) onion, cut in wedges

2 tablespoons (28 ml) olive oil

28 ounces (785 g) no-salt-added stewed tomatoes

¼ teaspoon cayenne pepper

¼ teaspoon black pepper

2 tablespoons (3 g) sugar substitute, such as Splenda

14 ounces (390 g) corned beef

In large pot, add sliced cabbage and ½ cup (120 ml) water. Steam 10 minutes. In large skillet, sauté onion in oil until clear. Add stewed tomatoes. Add cayenne pepper, black pepper, and sugar substitute. Cook 20 minutes. Pour over cabbage. Cook cabbage and tomato mixture 10 more minutes. Add corned beef and cook about 6 minutes longer or until cabbage is crisp-tender.

—
4 servings

Each with: 351 Calories (47% from Fat, 15% from Protein, 38% from Carb); 14 g Protein; 19 g Total Fat; 6 g Unsaturated Fat; 11 g Monounsaturated Fat; 1 g Polyunsaturated Fat; 35 g Carb; 8 g Fiber; 16 g Sugar; 176 mg Phosphorus; 158 mg Calcium; 1090 mg Sodium; 1011 mg Potassium; 621 IU Vitamin A; 0 mg ATE Vitamin E; 62 mg Vitamin C; 35 mg Cholesterol

Dinners: Pork

Everything I said in the introduction to the beef chapter also applies here. Pork can be very high in fat content or if you are careful can fit easily into your diet. About the only pork we buy are whole pork loins, which I grab when they are on sale and cut into chops, roasts, cubes, and grind up the end pieces to make sausage. Pork loin is great because it is naturally low in fat and what fat it does have can be easily trimmed off. And it can be used in almost any kind of recipe, as this chapter proves. There also are a few recipes here that call for ham. We don't eat ham very often because of the high sodium content, but it is an occasional treat. There is also one lamb stew recipe thrown in so you lamb lovers don't feel left out.

Italian Pork Chops

Here are Italian-style pork chops, cooked to a tender goodness in tomato sauce. There's enough sauce here to serve over both the pork and the pasta.

2 tablespoons (28 ml) olive oil

4 pork loin chops

1 cup (160 g) onion, chopped

1 cup (150 g) green bell pepper, chopped

½ teaspoon garlic, minced

2 cups (360 g) no-salt-added tomatoes

1 teaspoon Italian seasoning

¼ teaspoon black pepper

8 ounces (225 g) whole wheat spaghetti

1 pound (455 g) frozen Italian vegetable mix

In a large skillet, heat the oil and brown the pork chops for 2 to 3 minutes per side. Remove the chops from the skillet and cover to keep warm. Add the onion, green bell pepper, and garlic to the skillet and sauté for 3 to 5 minutes until tender and lightly browned. Stir in the tomatoes, Italian seasoning, and black pepper. Return the pork chops to the skillet; reduce the heat to low, cover, and simmer for about 30 minutes or until the chops are cooked through. Prepare pasta and vegetable mix according to package directions. Serve pork chops and pasta with sauce over both and vegetables on the side.

—

4 servings

Each with: 373 Calories (28% from Fat, 31% from Protein, 41% from Carb); 30 g Protein; 12 g Total Fat; 3 g Unsaturated Fat; 7 g Monounsaturated Fat; 2 g Polyunsaturated Fat; 40 g Carb; 8 g Fiber; 6 g Sugar; 372 mg Phosphorus; 100 mg Calcium; 120 mg Sodium; 976 mg Potassium; 5943 IU Vitamin A; 2 mg ATE Vitamin E; 33 mg Vitamin C; 64 mg Cholesterol

Touch of the South Bourbon Pork Chops

This is a real southern United States treat with a bourbon flavored pecan onion relish topping, but it's still healthy and low in calories thanks to the use of lean loin chops.

2 tablespoons (28 g) unsalted butter

2 cups (320 g) onion, sliced

2 ounces (28 ml) bourbon

¼ cup (28 g) pecans, toasted and sliced

2 tablespoons (5 g) sage leaves, minced

2 tablespoons (28 ml) olive oil

4 pork loin chops

4 cups (496 g) frozen green beans

Melt butter in skillet over medium-high heat. Add onion. Sauté 1 minute and then cover and reduce heat to medium low. Simmer 10 minutes. Stir onion, scraping bits from bottom of pan. Continue cooking onion, uncovered, until they become caramelized. Add bourbon. Cook for 2 to 3 minutes or until almost all liquid is evaporated. Transfer onion to a bowl. Stir in pecans and sage. Keep warm. Wipe out pan with a paper towel. Add oil to pan. Add chops to pan. Turn burner to medium heat. Cook chops until browned, about 5 minutes. Flip chops, cover pan, reduce heat to low, and cook for another 7 to 10 minutes. When ready to serve, top each chop with a helping of the onion pecan mixture. Serve with prepared green beans.

—

4 servings

Each with: 393 Calories (54% from Fat, 27% from Protein, 19% from Carb); 25 g Protein; 22 g Total Fat; 7 g Unsaturated Fat; 11 g Monounsaturated Fat; 3 g Polyunsaturated Fat; 18 g Carb; 6 g Fiber; 5 g Sugar; 306 mg Phosphorus; 95 mg Calcium; 62 mg Sodium; 760 mg Potassium; 1008 IU Vitamin A; 50 mg ATE Vitamin E; 24 mg Vitamin C; 79 mg Cholesterol

Pork and Squash Packets on the Grill

Pork, apples, and acorn squash wrapped in foil bake on the grill or in the oven for an easy meal and exceptional tenderness. The meal just says autumn in every way with its apples and winter squash, flavored with just a little brown sugar.

2 boneless pork loin chops, 1-inch (2.5 cm) thick

1 dash black pepper

3 cups (420 g) acorn squash, cut in ½-inch (1.3 cm) cubes

1 apple, cut in wedges

2 tablespoons (28 g) unsalted butter

2 tablespoons (2 g) brown sugar substitute, such as Splenda

Cut two 18 × 12-inch (46 × 30 cm) pieces of heavy foil; place pork chop in center of lower half of each piece of foil. Sprinkle with black pepper. Lay squash and apples on top of chop. Dot butter in center of each. Sprinkle with brown sugar substitute. Fold upper edge of foil over ingredients to meet bottom edge. Turn foil edges to form a ½-inch (1.3 cm) fold. Smooth fold. Double over again; press very tightly to seal, allowing room for expansion and heat circulation. Repeat folding and sealing at each end. Place packet on a baking sheet; bake at 425°F (220°C, or gas mark 7) or grill over medium heat for 25 to 30 minutes or until chops are done and vegetables are tender.

—
2 servings

Each with: 346 Calories (40% from Fat, 26% from Protein, 34% from Carb); 23 g Protein; 16 g Total Fat; 9 g Unsaturated Fat; 5 g Monounsaturated Fat; 1 g Polyunsaturated Fat; 30 g Carb; 4 g Fiber; 6 g Sugar; 306 mg Phosphorus; 89 mg Calcium; 59 mg Sodium; 1163 mg Potassium; 1157 IU Vitamin A; 97 mg ATE Vitamin E; 27 mg Vitamin C; 94 mg Cholesterol

Cowboy Skillet of Pork Chops and Beans

This is chuck wagon food from the American west. Or maybe it's just a great meal for a Saturday evening after working in the yard. This all in one pan meal will fill you up without filling you out thanks to lean pork loin, which cowboys probably never had.

6 boneless pork loin chops

1 tablespoon (15 ml) olive oil

1 cup (160 g) onion, chopped

1 cup (150 g) green bell pepper, chopped

½ teaspoon garlic, minced

½ cup (120 ml) low sodium chicken broth

½ cup (65 g) barbecue sauce

2 jalapeño peppers, chopped

4 cups (684 g) no-salt-added pinto beans, drained

In a large skillet, sear pork chops in oil until brown, about 5 minutes. Remove pork chops and place on plate. Add onion, green bell pepper, and garlic to skillet. Cook 10 minutes. Stir in broth, barbecue sauce, jalapeño pepper, and beans. Heat mixture to a boil. Return pork to skillet. Reduce heat. Cover and simmer 50 to 60 minutes, stirring sauce and turning chops occasionally until meat is fork-tender.

—
6 servings

Each with: 372 Calories (19% from Fat, 35% from Protein, 46% from Carb); 33 g Protein; 8 g Total Fat; 2 g Unsaturated Fat; 4 g Monounsaturated Fat; 1 g Polyunsaturated Fat; 43 g Carb; 10 g Fiber; 10 g Sugar; 393 mg Phosphorus; 71 mg Calcium; 273 mg Sodium; 813 mg Potassium; 137 IU Vitamin A; 2 mg ATE Vitamin E; 26 mg Vitamin C; 64 mg Cholesterol

Apple Cranberry Stuffed Pork Roast with Sweet Potatoes

When I made this, my wife wondered about going to the trouble of butterflying the roast, but the results were worth what turned out to be not a lot of effort.

FILLING

⅔ cup (160 ml) apple cider

¼ cup (60 ml) cider vinegar

½ cup (8 g) brown sugar substitute, such as Splenda

1 tablespoon (10 g) shallots, dried

1 cup (86 g) apples, dried

½ cup (60 g) dried cranberries

1 teaspoon ground ginger

½ teaspoon mustard seed

½ teaspoon allspice, ground

⅛ teaspoon cayenne pepper

PORK ROAST

2 pound (900 g) boneless pork loin roast

APPLE SWEET POTATO SIDE DISH

6 sweet potatoes, peeled and cubed

6 apples, peeled, cored and cubed

½ cup (120 ml) apple juice

½ teaspoon cinnamon

Simmer filling ingredients in medium saucepan over medium-high heat. Cover, reduce heat, and cook until apples are very soft, about 20 minutes. Strain through a fine-mesh sieve, reserving the liquid. Return liquid to saucepan and simmer over medium-high heat until reduced to ½ cup (120 ml), about 5 minutes. Remove from heat, set aside, and reserve as a glaze. Preheat oven to 350°F (180°C, or gas mark 4). Lay the roast down, fat side up. Insert the knife into the roast ½ inch (1.3 cm) horizontally from the bottom of the roast, along the long side of the roast. Make a long cut along the bottom of the roast, stopping ½ inch (1.3 cm) before the edge. Open up the roast and continue to cut through the thicker half of the roast, keeping ½ inch (1.3 cm) from the bottom. Repeat until the roast is an even ½- inch (1.3 cm) thickness all over when laid out. Spread out the filling on the roast, leaving a ½-inch (1.3 cm) border from the edges. Starting with the short side of the roast, roll it up very tightly. Secure with kitchen twine at 1-inch (2.5 cm) intervals. Place roast on a rack in a roasting pan and place in oven on the middle rack. Cook for 45 to 60 minutes. Brush with half of the glaze and cook for 5 minutes longer. Remove the roast from the oven. Cover with foil to rest and keep warm for 15 minutes before slicing. Slice into ½-inch (1.3 cm) wide pieces, removing the cooking twine as you cut the roast. Serve with remaining glaze. After putting roast in the oven, peel and cube the apples and sweet potatoes. Transfer to an 8-inch (20 cm) square baking dish. Combine the apple juice and cinnamon and pour over. Place in oven and allow to cook until roast is done.

—

8 servings

Each with: 366 Calories (20% from Fat, 30% from Protein, 51% from Carb); 27 g Protein; 8 g Total Fat; 3 g Saturated Fat; 3 g Monounsaturated Fat; 1 g Polyunsaturated Fat; 46 g Carb; 5 g Fiber; 27 g Sugar; 290 mg Phosphorus; 50 mg Calcium; 84 mg Sodium; 902 mg Potassium; 17 937 IU Vitamin A; 2 mg ATE Vitamin E; 20 mg Vitamin C; 62 mg Cholesterol

Greek Gods Pork Loin

A Mediterranean-style sauce makes these thin pork slices a little different meal. Low in fat with the pork loin and high in flavor, this meal is sure to be popular.

12 ounce (340 g) pork loin, cut into ¼-inch (6 mm) thick slices

⅛ teaspoon black pepper

2 teaspoons olive oil

1½ cups (240 g) onion, cut into thin wedges

1 cup (150 g) green bell pepper, cut into thin bite-size strips

½ cup (35 g) mushrooms, sliced

2 cloves garlic, minced

½ teaspoon dried oregano

⅓ cup (47 g) pimento stuffed olives, sliced

4 cups (628 g) couscous, cooked

4 cups (400 g) green beans

Spray a large skillet with nonstick vegetable oil spray: heat over medium-high heat. Season pork with black pepper. Cook half of the pork slices at a time in skillet for 2 to 3 minutes or until meat is browned and no longer pink in center, turning once. Remove from heat: keep warm. Add olive oil to skillet. Heat over medium-high heat. Cook onion, green bell pepper, mushrooms, garlic, and oregano in skillet about 4 minutes or until crisp-tender. Stir in olives; heat through. Serve vegetable mixture and pork slices over couscous with beans on the side.

—
4 servings

Each with: 374 Calories (15% from Fat, 29% from Protein, 56% from Carb); 27 g Protein; 6 g Total Fat; 2 g Unsaturated Fat; 3 g Monounsaturated Fat; 1 g Polyunsaturated Fat; 53 g Carb; 8 g Fiber; 5 g Sugar; 293 mg Phosphorus; 84 mg Calcium; 61 mg Sodium; 818 mg Potassium; 913 IU Vitamin A; 2 mg ATE Vitamin E; 53 mg Vitamin C; 54 mg Cholesterol

Glazed Pork Roast with Vegetables

I grill this when it's warm enough. If you want to do that, it's best to grill using indirect heat. Place a pan of water under the roast and mound the charcoal around it or grill on the side with no flame on a gas grill. Close the grill to hold in the heat and smoke.

¼ cup (85 g) honey

1 tablespoon (9 g) dry mustard

¼ cup (60 ml) white wine vinegar

1 teaspoon chili powder

2 pound (900 g) pork tenderloin

4 medium potatoes

2 cups (244 g) carrot, sliced

4 medium turnips

Mix together honey, mustard, vinegar, and chili powder. Trim any excess fat from pork roast. Brush with glaze. Place in roasting pan surrounded by vegetables. Roast at 350°F (180°C, or gas mark 4) until done, 1 to 1½ hours, brushing with additional glaze occasionally.

—
8 servings

Each with: 356 Calories (11% from Fat, 33% from Protein, 56% from Carb); 29 g Protein; 4 g Total Fat; 1 g Unsaturated Fat; 2 g Monounsaturated Fat; 1 g Polyunsaturated Fat; 50 g Carb; 6 g Fiber; 14 g Sugar; 400 mg Phosphorus; 74 mg Calcium; 156 mg Sodium; 1537 mg Potassium; 3968 IU Vitamin A; 2 mg ATE Vitamin E; 42 mg Vitamin C; 74 mg Cholesterol

Pork Roast with Apples and Potatoes and Other Good Stuff

A pork loin roast, cooked with apples and vegetables, makes a great looking as well as great tasting meal. And the loin cut is low in fat. This recipe makes enough for a large get together, but if you have a smaller family, the leftovers are also good.

¾ teaspoon black pepper

2 pound (900 g) pork loin roast

8 small onions, peeled but left whole

8 medium potatoes

2 cups carrot, cut in 2-inch (5 cm) pieces

8 apples, cored

2 cups (475 g) apple cider

Sprinkle black pepper over pork roast and place in roasting pan. Roast at 325°F (170°C, or gas mark 3) for 1 hour. Pour off fat. Place vegetables and apples in alternate positions around roast. Add cider and roast an additional 1 to 1½ hours, basting often. Skim off fat when done.

—
8 servings

Each with: 429 Calories (20% from Fat, 44% from Protein, 36% from Carb); 47 g Protein; 9 g Total Fat; 3 g Saturated Fat; 4 g Monounsaturated Fat; 1 g Polyunsaturated Fat; 39 g Carb; 4 g Fiber; 26 g Sugar; 530 mg Phosphorus; 76 mg Calcium; 137 mg Sodium; 1261 mg Potassium; 3927 IU Vitamin A; 4 mg ATE Vitamin E; 18 mg Vitamin C; 135 mg Cholesterol

Lechon Asado Roast Pork

Lechon asado is a Cuban pork disk. The original uses sour orange juice, but in this case we substitute a combination of lime and orange juice for this ingredient that is often difficult to find. Vegetables, including some nontraditional ones like cauliflower, cook around it for a tasty and healthy one pan oven meal.

1 tablespoon (10 g) garlic, minced

1 bay leaf, ground

½ teaspoon dried oregano

½ teaspoon ground cumin

1 tablespoon (15 ml) olive oil

3 pound (1⅓ kg) pork loin roast

½ teaspoon black pepper, fresh ground

¼ cup (60 ml) orange juice

¼ cup (60 ml) lime juice

¼ cup (60 ml) dry white wine

1½ cups (240 g) onion, sliced

5 medium potatoes, peeled and quartered

2 pounds (900 g) cauliflower florets, steamed until crisp-tender

Mash the garlic into a paste and then add the ground bay leaf, oregano, cumin, and olive oil and mix together. Rub this all over the roast. Place roast in a large glass dish and then sprinkle with black pepper and pour orange and lime juice and wine over. Scatter the onion over the roast and then wrap entire roast in plastic and refrigerate. Marinate at least one hour or overnight, turning several times. Heat oven to 350°F (180°C, or gas mark 4). Put the meat in a roasting pan, saving the marinade, and place in the oven. Cook for an hour. Turn roast over, add marinated onion and other vegetables, and reduce heat to 325°F (170°C, or gas mark 3). Baste frequently with the pan juices and continue cooking until done (30 to 35 minutes to the pound, 180°F [82°C] internal temperature). Add water or wine if necessary to keep from burning.

10 servings

Each with: 360 Calories (20% from Fat, 38% from Protein, 42% from Carb); 34 g Protein; 8 g Total Fat; 2 g Unsaturated Fat; 4 g Monounsaturated Fat; 1 g Polyunsaturated Fat; 37 g Carb; 6 g Fiber; 4 g Sugar; 449 mg Phosphorus; 61 mg Calcium; 96 mg Sodium; 1537 mg Potassium; 47 IU Vitamin A; 3 mg ATE Vitamin E; 83 mg Vitamin C; 86 mg Cholesterol

Pork Tenderloin with Cabbage and Apple Slaw

Tender lean pork tenderloin is simply prepared and teamed with a slaw containing Napa cabbage and apple. The potatoes here show one of the tricks of low calorie cooking. By slicing them thinly, each serving contains more slices and looks bigger, but we hold down the calories.

3 tablespoons (45 ml) olive oil, divided

2½ pound (1.1 kg) pork tenderloin

¼ teaspoon black pepper

2 tablespoons (28 ml) rice vinegar

1 tablespoon (20 g) honey

1 pound (455 g) Napa cabbage, cored, and thinly sliced

1 apple, cut into thin wedges

¼ cup (4 g) fresh cilantro

2 red potatoes, sliced ¼-inch (6 mm) thick and boiled

Preheat oven to 400°F (200°C, or gas mark 6). Heat 1 tablespoon (15 ml) of the oil in a large ovenproof skillet over medium-high heat. Season the pork with black pepper and cook, turning occasionally, until browned, 6 to 8 minutes. Transfer the skillet to the oven and roast until the pork is cooked through, 12 to 14 minutes. Let rest at least 5 minutes before slicing. Meanwhile, in a large bowl, combine the vinegar, honey, and remaining 2 tablespoons (28 ml) of oil. Add the cabbage and apples and toss. Let sit for at least 5 minutes, tossing occasionally. Fold in the cilantro and serve with the pork and potatoes.

6 servings

Each with: 406 Calories (30% from Fat, 43% from Protein, 27% from Carb); 43 g Protein; 14 g Total Fat; 3 g Unsaturated Fat; 8 g Monounsaturated Fat; 1 g Polyunsaturated Fat; 27 g Carb; 2 g Fiber; 7 g Sugar; 521 mg Phosphorus; 47 mg Calcium; 112 mg Sodium; 1354 mg Potassium; 347 IU Vitamin A; 4 mg ATE Vitamin E; 30 mg Vitamin C; 123 mg Cholesterol

Sweet and Sour Pork Tenderloin

Hot, slightly sweet ginger gives the sauce a little bite. Fruit and vegetables add nutrition. This is a very tasty way to do pork tenderloin, and one that will not remind you that you are trying to lose weight.

2 tablespoons (28 ml) olive oil

1 tablespoon (6 g) fresh ginger, minced

½ teaspoon garlic, smashed

1 green bell pepper, cored, seeded, and cut in strips

1 pound (455 g) pork tenderloin, in 1-inch (2.5 cm) cubes

1 tablespoon (8 g) all purpose flour

1 cup (235 ml) low sodium beef broth

1 tablespoon (16 g) no-salt-added tomato paste

1 tablespoon (15 ml) low sodium soy sauce

1 tablespoon (15 ml) lemon juice

3 tablespoons (48 g) mango chutney

1 cup (165 g) pineapple chunks, in juice

2 cups (390 g) brown rice, cooked

Heat 1 tablespoon (15 ml) oil in medium nonstick skillet. Add ginger root, garlic, and green bell pepper and sauté over medium heat 5 minutes. Add remaining 1 tablespoon (15 ml) oil to skillet. Dust pork cubes with flour and add to skillet. Brown pork over high heat, turning to brown evenly. Pour in beef broth and stir up any browned bits in the skillet. Add tomato paste, soy sauce, lemon juice, and chutney. Stir mixture well. Cover skillet and simmer 10 minutes. Mixture will thicken. Stir in pineapple. Cover and simmer another 5 minutes. Serve over hot cooked rice.

—

4 servings

Each with: 384 Calories (28% from Fat, 29% from Protein, 43% from Carb); 28 g Protein; 12 g Total Fat; 3 g Unsaturated Fat; 7 g Monounsaturated Fat; 1 g Polyunsaturated Fat; 41 g Carb; 4 g Fiber; 6 g Sugar; 362 mg Phosphorus; 37 mg Calcium; 235 mg Sodium; 755 mg Potassium; 338 IU Vitamin A; 2 mg ATE Vitamin E; 39 mg Vitamin C; 74 mg Cholesterol

Pork Stroganoff with All the Trimmings

Even though beef is more traditional for stroganoff, this works well too. At least around here, you can buy a boneless pork loin for less than ground beef or any other beef cut for that matter. And it's a great deal nutritionally since it's so low in fat. So you can still have the noodles and broccoli.

1½ pound (680 g) pork loin, cubed

1 tablespoon (15 ml) olive oil

½ cup (80 g) onion, chopped

1 cup (235 ml) low sodium beef broth

8 ounces (225 g) mushrooms, sliced

¼ teaspoon garlic powder

1 teaspoon dill weed

⅛ teaspoon black pepper

½ cup (115 g) fat-free sour cream

¼ cup (60 ml) white wine

3 tablespoons (24 g) all purpose flour

2 cups (320 g) egg noodles, cooked

4 cups (284 g) broccoli florets, steamed until crisp-tender

In a skillet, brown the meat in the oil. Add the onion and cook until softened. Transfer to slow cooker. Combine broth, mushrooms, and spices. Pour over meat mixture. Cook on low for 8 to 10 hours or on high for 5 to 6 hours. Turn heat to high. Stir together sour cream, wine, and flour. Add to cooker. Cook until sauce is thickened, about 15 to 20 minutes. Serve over noodles with broccoli on the side.

—

6 servings

Each with: 416 Calories (48% from Fat, 29% from Protein, 23% from Carb); 30 g Protein; 22 g Total Fat; 8 g Unsaturated Fat; 10 g Monounsaturated Fat; 2 g Polyunsaturated Fat; 24 g Carb; 3 g Fiber; 3 g Sugar; 361 mg Phosphorus; 72 mg Calcium; 105 mg Sodium; 841 mg Potassium; 491 IU Vitamin A; 26 mg ATE Vitamin E; 55 mg Vitamin C; 94 mg Cholesterol

Pork and Chickpea Stir-Fry

This is a stir-fry in the cooking method but not in the usual ingredients. It's a simple meal that's quickly cooked, full of nutrition, and great tasting.

1 pound (455 g) boneless pork loin chops, cut into 1½-inch (3.8 cm) thick strips

¼ cup (25 g) green onion, with tops, sliced

½ teaspoon garlic, crushed

2 teaspoons olive oil

2 cups (142 g) broccoli florets

3 cups (720 g) chickpeas, drained and rinsed

¼ cup (60 ml) low sodium beef broth

Stir-fry pork, green onion, and garlic in oil in wok or large skillet over high heat until pork is browned, 3 to 5 minutes. Add broccoli and stir-fry 2 to 3 minutes. Add chickpeas and broth and cook, covered, over medium heat until broccoli is crisp-tender, 3 to 4 minutes.

—
4 servings

Each with: 380 Calories (24% from Fat, 38% from Protein, 38% from Carb); 36 g Protein; 10 g Total Fat; 2 g Unsaturated Fat; 5 g Monounsaturated Fat; 2 g Polyunsaturated Fat; 36 g Carb; 10 g Fiber; 6 g Sugar; 482 mg Phosphorus; 98 mg Calcium; 86 mg Sodium; 920 mg Potassium; 1168 IU Vitamin A; 2 mg ATE Vitamin E; 37 mg Vitamin C; 71 mg Cholesterol

Stuffed Acorn Squash

This acorn squash stuffed with a ground pork mixture is a favorite around our house.

1 acorn squash, about 1 pound (455 g)

6 ounces (170 g) ground pork

¼ cup (25 g) celery, chopped

½ cup (80 g) onion, chopped

¼ teaspoon curry powder

¼ teaspoon cinnamon

½ cup (123 g) applesauce, unsweetened

1 slice whole wheat bread, cubed

Spray a 10 × 6 × 2-inch (25 × 15 × 5 cm) baking dish with nonstick vegetable oil spray. Halve squash; discard seeds. Place squash, cut side down, in baking dish. Bake, uncovered, in 350°F (180°C, or gas mark 4) oven for 50 minutes. Meanwhile, for stuffing, in a skillet, cook pork, celery, and onion until meat is no longer pink and vegetables are tender. Drain fat. Stir in curry powder and cinnamon; cook 1 minute more. Stir in applesauce and bread cubes. Turn squash cut side up in dish. Place stuffing in squash halves. Bake uncovered, 20 minutes more.

—
2 servings

Each with: 389 Calories (42% from Fat, 18% from Protein, 40% from Carb); 18 g Protein; 19 g Total Fat; 7 g Saturated Fat; 8 g Monounsaturated Fat; 2 g Polyunsaturated Fat; 40 g Carb; 6 g Fiber; 9 g Sugar; 265 mg Phosphorus; 118 mg Calcium; 135 mg Sodium; 1165 mg Potassium; 886 IU Vitamin A; 2 mg ATE Vitamin E; 28 mg Vitamin C; 61 mg Cholesterol

TIP:

You could reduce the number of calories and amount of fat by using ground turkey.

Cabbage Casserole

Ground turkey and sausage mix with brown rice and vegetables for an easy casserole that is full of flavor and nutrition without being full of calories.

½ pound (225 g) ground turkey

½ pound (225 g) sausage, cut into small pieces

2 cups (360 g) no-salt-added tomatoes

1 cup (160 g) onion, chopped

1 cup (190 g) brown rice, uncooked

1 tablespoon (8 g) chili powder

1 teaspoon garlic powder

1 cup (150 g) green bell pepper, chopped

4 cups (360 g) cabbage, shredded

¼ cup (60 ml) egg substitute

Mix all ingredients together in covered roasting pan. Bake at 350°F (180°C, or gas mark 4) for approximately 1½ hours. Stir a couple of times.

—
4 servings

Each with: 424 Calories (25% from Fat, 25% from Protein, 50% from Carb); 27 g Protein; 12 g Total Fat; 4 g Unsaturated Fat; 5 g Monounsaturated Fat; 2 g Polyunsaturated Fat; 54 g Carb; 7 g Fiber; 10 g Sugar; 375 mg Phosphorus; 131 mg Calcium; 352 mg Sodium; 1077 mg Potassium; 1060 IU Vitamin A; 0 mg ATE Vitamin E; 80 mg Vitamin C; 56 mg Cholesterol

Easy Does It Pork Stew

Easy to make in the slow cooker and chock full of vegetables, this is the kind of stew I'd want even if I weren't being careful about my diet.

1 pound (455 g) ground pork

1 cup (160 g) onion, chopped

1 cup (122 g) carrot, sliced

1 cup (150 g) turnip, diced

½ cup (50 g) celery, sliced

1 medium sweet potato, cubed and peeled

½ teaspoon dried rosemary

1 cup (235 ml) low sodium beef broth

Place meat and onion in nonstick skillet. Brown on stove top. Place drained meat and onion into slow cooker. Add remaining ingredients. Cover and cook on low for 6 to 8 hours.

—
4 servings

Each with: 372 Calories (59% from Fat, 23% from Protein, 18% from Carb); 21 g Protein; 24 g Total Fat; 9 g Unsaturated Fat; 11 g Monounsaturated Fat; 2 g Polyunsaturated Fat; 16 g Carb; 3 g Fiber; 7 g Sugar; 253 mg Phosphorus; 65 mg Calcium; 166 mg Sodium; 706 mg Potassium; 9883 IU Vitamin A; 2 mg ATE Vitamin E; 17 mg Vitamin C; 82 mg Cholesterol

Chinese Shredded Pork and Cabbage

If you replace the large amount of white rice with reasonable amounts of brown and feature lean meat and lots of vegetables, you can get a meal like this that tastes great, fills you up, and provides excellent nutrition.

1 pound (455 g) pork loin roast

4 tablespoons (60 ml) olive oil

2 cups (180 g) cabbage, shredded

1 cup (110 g) carrot, shredded

1 cup (160 g) onion, cut in strips

½ teaspoon oriental seasoning

¼ cup (60 ml) low sodium soy sauce

2 cups (390 g) cooked brown rice

Slice pork thinly and then shred the strips. Heat 2 tablespoons (28 ml) of the oil in a wok or heavy skillet. Stir-fry the pork until cooked through. Remove from wok. Add the other two tablespoons (28 ml) of oil and stir-fry the vegetables until crisp-tender. Return the pork to the wok. Add the seasoning and soy sauce. Heat through. Serve over rice.

—

4 servings

Each with: 421 Calories (41% from Fat, 27% from Protein, 32% from Carb); 28 g Protein; 19 g Total Fat; 4 g Saturated Fat; 12 g Monounsaturated Fat; 2 g Polyunsaturated Fat; 33 g Carb; 4 g Fiber; 3 g Sugar; 370 mg Phosphorus; 63 mg Calcium; 621 mg Sodium; 772 mg Potassium; 3937 IU Vitamin A; 2 mg ATE Vitamin E; 23 mg Vitamin C; 71 mg Cholesterol

Chinese Pork Stir-Fry

This is a fairly traditional Chinese style stir-fry, but it has a few more vegetables and a bit less rice to up the nutrition and lower the calories.

1 pound (455 g) pork loin

3 tablespoons (45 ml) olive oil

2 cups (180 g) cabbage, shredded

½ cup (55 g) carrot, shredded

1½ cups (107 g) broccoli florets

1 cup (160 g) onion, cut in strips

¼ cup (60 ml) low sodium soy sauce

½ teaspoon oriental seasoning

2 cups (390 g) brown rice, cooked

Slice pork thinly and then shred the strips. Heat 2 tablespoons (28 ml) of the oil in a wok or heavy skillet. Stir-fry the pork until cooked through. Remove from wok. Add the other tablespoon (15 ml) of oil and stir-fry the vegetables until crisp-tender. Return the pork to the wok. Add the seasoning and soy sauce. Heat through. Serve over rice.

—

4 servings

Each with: 394 Calories (36% from Fat, 29% from Protein, 34% from Carb); 29 g Protein; 16 g Total Fat; 3 g Unsaturated Fat; 10 g Monounsaturated Fat; 2 g Polyunsaturated Fat; 34 g Carb; 4 g Fiber; 4 g Sugar; 384 mg Phosphorus; 75 mg Calcium; 619 mg Sodium; 831 mg Potassium; 2842 IU Vitamin A; 2 mg ATE Vitamin E; 44 mg Vitamin C; 71 mg Cholesterol

Old World Smoked Sausage Stew

This is the kind of meal I imagine my ancestors in Germany eating. It's a nice hearty stew of smoked sausage and beans that will both fill and warm you. In this version, we use turkey kielbasa, which helps to hold down the fat and calories, and there are plenty of vegetables to make it a meal in a bowl.

1 cup (160 g) onion, chopped

1 pound (455 g) turkey kielbasa, thinly sliced

2 tablespoons (28 ml) olive oil

30 ounces (840 g) great northern beans, no-salt-added, undrained

16 ounces (455 g) no-salt-added tomato sauce

4 ounces (115 g) diced green chilies

1 cup (122 g) carrot, thinly sliced

½ cup (75 g) green bell pepper, chopped

2 medium potatoes, diced

¼ teaspoon Italian seasoning

½ teaspoon dried thyme

¼ teaspoon black pepper

Sauté onion and kielbasa in oil in skillet until onions are soft. Transfer onions and kielbasa to slow cooker. Add all remaining ingredients to cooker and stir together well. Cover. Cook on low for 8 to 10 hours or until vegetables are tender.

—
8 servings

Each with: 393 Calories (32% from Fat, 19% from Protein, 50% from Carb); 18 g Protein; 14 g Total Fat; 4 g Unsaturated Fat; 7 g Monounsaturated Fat; 2 g Polyunsaturated Fat; 50 g Carb; 9 g Fiber; 4 g Sugar; 231 mg Phosphorus; 95 mg Calcium; 765 mg Sodium; 1109 mg Potassium; 2188 IU Vitamin A; 0 mg ATE Vitamin E; 41 mg Vitamin C; 40 mg Cholesterol

Full of Goodness Split Pea Soup with Ham

This is a little more than your usual split pea soup, with extra generous helpings of vegetables. Yet with all that taste and nutrition and the ability to fill you up and hold you over to the next meal, it still has less than 350 calories.

1 pound (455 g) ham, chopped

6 cups (1.4 L) water

1 pound (455 g) split peas

2 medium potatoes, peeled and diced

2½ cups (305 g) carrot, sliced

1½ cups (240 g) onion, chopped

1 cup (100 g) celery, chopped

½ teaspoon marjoram

¼ teaspoon black pepper

Place ham in slow cooker. Stir in water, peas, potatoes, carrot, onion, celery, marjoram, and black pepper. Cover and cook on low for 10 to 12 hours. Before serving, stir mixture.

—

6 servings

Each with: 346 Calories (18% from Fat, 29% from Protein, 53% from Carb); 25 g Protein; 7 g Total Fat; 2 g Unsaturated Fat; 3 g Monounsaturated Fat; 1 g Polyunsaturated Fat; 46 g Carb; 11 g Fiber; 8 g Sugar; 351 mg Phosphorus; 68 mg Calcium; 875 mg Sodium; 1380 mg Potassium; 6532 IU Vitamin A; 0 mg ATE Vitamin E; 31 mg Vitamin C; 31 mg Cholesterol

Pasta with Ham and Vegetables

This is a great pasta dish that can be eaten however you like it, hot, warm, or cold. Lots of zucchini and a little wine add interest, and spinach ups the nutrition index.

8 ounces (225 g) whole wheat pasta

4 tablespoons (60 ml) olive oil

½ pound (225 g) ham

6 cups (720 g) zucchini, sliced

1 cup (160 g) onion, sliced

½ cup (120 ml) white wine

6 ounces (170 g) spinach

Cook pasta according to directions. Add olive oil to a large nonstick pan. Add chopped ham and cook for about 5 minutes or until desired crispness. Add zucchini and onion to the pan with ham and oil and cook for about 10 more minutes, stirring occasionally until squash is golden brown. Add wine and cook about 5 more minutes. When done, add pasta and spinach and cook long enough for spinach to wilt.

—

4 servings

Each with: 361 Calories (48% from Fat, 21% from Protein, 31% from Carb); 19 g Protein; 19 g Total Fat; 4 g Unsaturated Fat; 12 g Monounsaturated Fat; 2 g Polyunsaturated Fat; 27 g Carb; 5 g Fiber; 6 g Sugar; 282 mg Phosphorus; 94 mg Calcium; 663 mg Sodium; 1030 mg Potassium; 4362 IU Vitamin A; 0 mg ATE Vitamin E; 46 mg Vitamin C; 23 mg Cholesterol

Ham Stuffed Eggplant

Ham may seem like an unusual meat to stuff eggplant with, but their flavors complement each other nicely. Tomatoes and other vegetables make this not just a filling meal, but one full of nutrition.

2 eggplants, each about 1 pound (455 g)

¼ cup (60 ml) olive oil

½ cup (80 g) onion, finely chopped

½ cup (50 g) scallions, finely chopped, including 3 inches (7.5 cm) of the green

1½ teaspoons garlic, minced

1 cup (180 g) no-salt-added tomatoes

1 teaspoon dried thyme

¼ teaspoon cayenne pepper

¼ teaspoon black pepper

½ pound (225 g) ham, finely ground

1½ cups (175 g) bread crumbs

¼ cup (15 g) fresh parsley, finely chopped

Cut the eggplants in half lengthwise and with a spoon, hollow out the center of each half to make a boat-like shell about ¼-inch (6 mm) thick. Finely chop the eggplant pulp and set aside. In a heavy skillet, heat the olive oil over moderate heat. Add the eggplant shells and turn them about with tongs until they are moistened on all sides. Then cover the skillet tightly and cook over moderate heat for 5 or 6 minutes. Turn the shells over and continue to cook, still tightly covered, for 5 minutes longer or until they are somewhat soft to the touch. Invert the shells on paper towels to drain and arrange them cut side up in a baking dish large enough to hold them snugly in one layer. Preheat the oven to 400°F (200°C, or gas mark 6). Add the onion, scallions, and garlic to the skillet and stirring frequently, cook for 5 minutes or until they are soft but not brown. Add the reserved chopped eggplant pulp, the tomatoes, thyme, cayenne pepper, and black pepper and stirring frequently, cook until most of the liquid in the pan evaporates and the mixture is thick enough to hold. Remove the skillet from the heat and stir in the ham, half of the bread crumbs, and the parsley. Spoon the filling into the eggplant shells, dividing it equally among them and mounding it slightly in the centers. Sprinkle shells with the remaining bread crumbs. Bake for 15 minutes or until the shells are tender and the filling lightly browned.

—
4 servings

Each with: 403 Calories (46% from Fat, 18% from Protein, 36% from Carb); 19 g Protein; 21 g Total Fat; 4 g Unsaturated Fat; 13 g Monounsaturated Fat; 3 g Polyunsaturated Fat; 36 g Carb; 3 g Fiber; 6 g Sugar; 219 mg Phosphorus; 123 mg Calcium; 914 mg Sodium; 518 mg Potassium; 576 IU Vitamin A; 0 mg ATE Vitamin E; 18 mg Vitamin C; 23 mg Cholesterol

Full Meal, Full You, Barley Salad

This makes a cool and crunchy salad with a vinaigrette dressing. Ham and barley add substance, as well as flavor.

1 cup (184 g) cooked
pearl barley

½ cup (62 g) water chestnuts,
drained, sliced

1 cup (100 g) celery, chopped

1 cup (150 g) green bell
pepper, chopped

⅓ cup (64 g) pimento

¼ cup (40 g) onion, chopped

1 cup (150 g) ham, cubed

1 tablespoon (6 g)
Italian seasoning

¼ cup (6 g) sugar substitute,
such as Splenda

¼ cup (60 ml) olive oil

¼ cup (60 ml) red wine vinegar

4 cups (228 g) mixed greens

Mix together cooked barley, water chestnuts, celery, green bell pepper, pimentos, onion, and ham. Cover and chill. In a screw-top jar, combine remaining ingredients except lettuce. Cover and shake well. Pour over salad and stir to mix just before serving. Place lettuce on plate and spoon salad on top.

—

4 servings

Each with: 385 Calories (40% from Fat, 15% from Protein, 45% from Carb); 15 g Protein; 18 g Total Fat; 3 g Saturated Fat; 12 g Monounsaturated Fat; 2 g Polyunsaturated Fat; 45 g Carb; 11 g Fiber; 5 g Sugar; 244 mg Phosphorus; 62 mg Calcium; 415 mg Sodium; 715 mg Potassium; 937 IU Vitamin A; 0 mg ATE Vitamin E; 48 mg Vitamin C; 14 mg Cholesterol

TIP:

Leave out the ham and serve with a piece of grilled meat.

You Can Have a Little Lamb and Vegetable Stew

Lamb is often high in fat and calories. But if you are careful to pick a lean cut like an arm steak and trim the fat, you can still have it occasionally. This stew is rich in vegetables, which don't add that many calories but fill you up and keep you from getting hungry soon after eating.

2 tablespoons (28 ml) olive oil

1 pound (455 g) lamb steaks, bones removed and meat cut into 2-inch (5 cm) pieces

½ teaspoon black pepper

1 cup (122 g) carrot, cut into 3-inch (7.5 cm) sticks

1 cup (160 g) onion, sliced

1 tablespoon (8 g) all purpose flour

½ cup (60 ml) dry white wine

2 cups (475 ml) low sodium chicken broth

2 cups (360 g) no-salt-added tomatoes, drained

4 ounces (115 g) green beans, cut into small pieces

1 cup (60 g) fresh parsley, chopped

Heat 1 tablespoon (15 ml) of the oil in a large pot over medium-high heat. Season the lamb with black pepper. Cook, turning occasionally, until medium-rare, 6 to 8 minutes; transfer to a plate. Add the carrot, onion, and the remaining oil to the pot. Cook until beginning to soften, 3 to 4 minutes. Add the flour and cook for 1 minute. Add the wine and scrape up any brown bits. Add the broth, tomatoes, and green beans. Simmer until the vegetables are tender, 8 to 10 minutes. Stir in the lamb and parsley.

—
4 servings

Each with: 381 Calories (58% from Fat, 22% from Protein, 20% from Carb); 20 g Protein; 24 g Total Fat; 8 g Unsaturated Fat; 12 g Monounsaturated Fat; 2 g Polyunsaturated Fat; 19 g Carb; 4 g Fiber; 7 g Sugar; 245 mg Phosphorus; 107 mg Calcium; 135 mg Sodium; 915 mg Potassium; 5470 IU Vitamin A; 0 mg ATE Vitamin E; 46 mg Vitamin C; 60 mg Cholesterol

Dinners: Fish and Seafood

Fish and seafood are great choices for those people looking to lose a little weight and still eat healthy food. They are generally low in calories, and they contain many valuable nutrients like omega-3 fatty acids. Fortunately, it's not difficult to create great recipes using fish and seafood. This chapter contains some of our favorites.

Oven Fried Fish

Nicely spiced fish is fried up in the oven with minimum fat.

2 tablespoons (28 g) unsalted butter, melted

1 tablespoon (15 ml) lemon juice

¼ teaspoon black pepper

¼ teaspoon paprika

¼ teaspoon dried basil

⅛ teaspoon garlic powder

1 pound (455 g) flounder

¼ cup (30 g) bread crumbs

2 tablespoons (28 ml) oil

2 medium potatoes

Combine butter, lemon juice, black pepper, paprika, basil, and garlic. Dredge fish in mixture and roll in bread crumbs. Spread oil in shallow baking dish and arrange fish in one layer. Spoon remaining mixture over fish. Cut potatoes into thin wedges and place on baking sheet. Spray with nonstick vegetable oil spray. Bake both uncovered at 475°F (240°C, or gas mark 9) for 15 minutes or until fish flakes easily with fork.

4 servings

Each with: 388 Calories (34% from Fat, 27% from Protein, 39% from Carb); 26 g Protein; 14 g Total Fat; 5 g Unsaturated Fat; 3 g Monounsaturated Fat; 5 g Polyunsaturated Fat; 37 g Carb; 4 g Fiber; 1 g Sugar; 329 mg Phosphorus; 63 mg Calcium; 154 mg Sodium; 1257 mg Potassium; 316 IU Vitamin A; 59 mg ATE Vitamin E; 23 mg Vitamin C; 70 mg Cholesterol

TIP:

Sprinkle the potatoes with garlic, black pepper, paprika, or other spices to suit your taste.

Not Your Mama's Tuna Casserole

This is a variation on the traditional tuna casserole. Brown rice contains more nutrients than the typical egg noodles, and yogurt provides flavor and creaminess. Plus extra vegetables add even more nutrition.

1¼ cup (238 g) brown rice, uncooked

3 cups (700 g) water

1 cup (100 g) chopped celery

½ cup (80 g) onion, finely diced

½ cup (115 g) plain fat-free yogurt

1 cup (235 ml) skim milk

1 cup (150 g) red bell pepper, chopped

½ teaspoon dried tarragon

14 ounces (390 g) tuna, water packed, drained

1½ cups (107 g) broccoli florets

20 ounces (570 g) frozen peas, thawed

¾ cup (86 g) low fat cheddar cheese, shredded

Combine rice and water in large saucepan. Bring to a boil. Reduce heat, cover, and cook 35 minutes. Remove from heat. Add celery, onion, yogurt, and skim milk. Add red bell pepper and tarragon; mix well. Add flaked tuna, broccoli, and thawed peas; mix well. Turn into 2-quart (1.9 L) casserole. Bake at 350°F (180°C, or gas mark 4) for 30 minutes. Top with shredded cheese.

6 servings

Each with: 372 Calories (8% from Fat, 35% from Protein, 56% from Carb); 33 g Protein; 3 g Total Fat; 1 g Saturated Fat; 1 g Monounsaturated Fat; 1 g Polyunsaturated Fat; 52 g Carb; 8 g Fiber; 4 g Sugar; 509 mg Phosphorus; 233 mg Calcium; 699 mg Sodium; 734 mg Potassium; 1803 IU Vitamin A; 47 mg ATE Vitamin E; 78 mg Vitamin C; 25 mg Cholesterol

More Like Your Mama's Tuna Casserole (Only Better and Easier)

Here's a fairly traditional tuna noodle casserole, with added vegetables, that cooks in the slow cooker.

16 ounces (455 g) tuna, water packed

20 ounces (570 g) low sodium cream of mushroom soup

1 cup (235 ml) skim milk

2 tablespoons (8 g) fresh parsley, chopped

8 ounces (225 g) mushrooms, sliced

16 ounces (455 g) frozen mixed vegetables, thawed

16 ounces (455 g) frozen broccoli, carrot and cauliflower, thawed

10 ounces (280 g) egg noodles, cooked and drained

¼ cup (23 g) sliced almonds, toasted

Combine tuna, soup, skim milk, parsley, and vegetables. Fold in noodles. Pour into greased slow cooker. Top with almonds. Cover. Cook on low for 7 to 9 hours or on high for 3 to 4 hours.

—

6 servings

Each with: 364 Calories (19% from Fat, 31% from Protein, 50% from Carb); 29 g Protein; 8 g Total Fat; 2 g Saturated Fat; 3 g Monounsaturated Fat; 2 g Polyunsaturated Fat; 45 g Carb; 11 g Fiber; 7 g Sugar; 433 mg Phosphorus; 136 mg Calcium; 481 mg Sodium; 1045 mg Potassium; 6705 IU Vitamin A; 31 mg ATE Vitamin E; 8 mg Vitamin C; 35 mg Cholesterol

Fish and Wine Sauced Pasta

This makes a simple but flavorful sauce that is particularly good with whole wheat pasta. And the meal gets a great nutritional bonus both from the fish and the generous serving of broccoli on the side.

¼ cup (60 ml) olive oil

12 ounces (340 g) salmon fillets, cubed

12 ounces (340 g) fish fillets, cubed

1 teaspoon minced garlic

½ cup (120 ml) white wine

½ teaspoon dried oregano

½ teaspoon dried rosemary

1 teaspoon dried parsley

1 tablespoon (10 g) minced onion

12 ounces (340 g) whole wheat spaghetti

6 cups (426 g) broccoli florets, steamed until crisp-tender

Heat oil in a heavy skillet. Add fish and garlic and sauté for a minute or two until nearly cooked through. Add wine, minced onion, and spices and continue cooking until sauce has been reduced to about half. Serve over pasta with broccoli.

—

6 servings

Each with: 370 Calories (42% from Fat, 34% from Protein, 24% from Carb); 30 g Protein; 17 g Total Fat; 3 g Unsaturated Fat; 9 g Monounsaturated Fat; 4 g Polyunsaturated Fat; 22 g Carb; 4 g Fiber; 2 g Sugar; 404 mg Phosphorus; 141 mg Calcium; 120 mg Sodium; 741 mg Potassium; 662 IU Vitamin A; 16 mg ATE Vitamin E; 82 mg Vitamin C; 64 mg Cholesterol

Creamed Fish Fillets with Shrimp Sauce

Fish is poached in milk and then covered with a cheesy sauce containing shrimp in this recipe. It is the sort of thing to pull out and serve to company and then surprise them with the fact that it is *diet* food.

1 pound (455 g) cod, or other white fish

¼ cup (40 g) onion, minced

1½ cups (355 ml) skim milk

2 tablespoons (28 g) butter or margarine

2 tablespoons (16 g) all purpose flour

⅛ teaspoon black pepper

¼ cup (25 g) Parmesan cheese, grated

6 ounces (170 g) shrimp, cleaned, cooked, and chopped

2 tablespoons (28 ml) sherry

1 tablespoon (4 g) fresh parsley, minced

2 cups (390 g) brown rice, cooked

Slice fish in thin pieces. Place in greased baking dish and sprinkle with minced onion. Pour skim milk over fish. Bake in 400°F (200°C, or gas mark 6) oven until done. Fish may take anywhere from 15 to 30 minutes to bake, depending on thickness. When it is easily flaked with fork, it is ready. Meanwhile, melt butter in sauce pan; stir in flour and black pepper. When fish is done, remove from oven and turn up heat to 450°F (230°C, or gas mark 8). Pour milk out of fish pan and stir into butter mixture. Cook sauce, while stirring, until smooth and thickened. Add cheese and stir until melted. Add shrimp; heat. Stir in sherry. Pour sauce over fish; sprinkle with parsley and put back in oven to bake for 5 minutes or until very lightly browned. Serve over rice.

—
4 servings

Each with: 393 Calories (24% from Fat, 40% from Protein, 36% from Carb); 38 g Protein; 10 g Total Fat; 5 g Unsaturated Fat; 3 g Monounsaturated Fat; 1 g Polyunsaturated Fat; 34 g Carb; 2 g Fiber; 1 g Sugar; 551 mg Phosphorus; 258 mg Calcium; 318 mg Sodium; 832 mg Potassium; 596 IU Vitamin A; 148 mg ATE Vitamin E; 5 mg Vitamin C; 136 mg Cholesterol

Catfish Parmesan

Oven baked fish and potatoes are crunchy and full of flavor but not full of fat and calories.

2½ pounds (1.1 kg) catfish fillets, fresh or frozen

1 cup (115 g) bread crumbs

¾ cup (75 g) Parmesan cheese, grated

1 teaspoon paprika

½ teaspoon dried oregano

¼ teaspoon dried basil

½ teaspoon black pepper

2 tablespoons (28 g) unsalted butter, melted

2 medium potatoes, cut in wedges

1 lemon, cut in wedges

¼ cup (15 g) fresh parsley, chopped

20 ounces (570 g) green beans

Pat fish dry. Combine bread crumbs, cheese, and seasonings; stir well. Dip catfish in butter and roll each in crumb mixture. Arrange fish on baking sheet sprayed with nonstick vegetable oil spray. Place potato wedges around fish. Bake at 375°F (190°C, or gas mark 5) about 25 minutes or until fish flakes easily when tested with a fork. Garnish with lemon wedges and parsley. Serve with potatoes and green beans.

—

8 servings

Each with: 410 Calories (38% from Fat, 30% from Protein, 32% from Carb); 31 g Protein; 17 g Total Fat; 6 g Unsaturated Fat; 7 g Monounsaturated Fat; 3 g Polyunsaturated Fat; 32 g Carb; 5 g Fiber; 2 g Sugar; 462 mg Phosphorus; 191 mg Calcium; 330 mg Sodium; 1062 mg Potassium; 1179 IU Vitamin A; 56 mg ATE Vitamin E; 31 mg Vitamin C; 82 mg Cholesterol

Tuna Broccoli Rollups

These are sort of tuna enchiladas, full of a creamy tuna and broccoli mixture that tastes as good as it is good for you.

¼ cup (60 ml) skim milk

1 tablespoon (15 ml) lemon juice

1 can (10¾ ounces, or 305 g) low sodium cream of mushroom soup

7 ounces (200 g) tuna, drained

10 ounces (280 g) broccoli, thawed and drained

4 ounces (115 g) low fat cheddar cheese, shredded, divided

3 whole wheat tortillas, 8-inch (20 cm)

1 cup (180 g) tomato, chopped

Combine skim milk, lemon juice, and mushroom soup. Mix tuna, broccoli, and ½ of cheese in separate bowl. Stir ¾ cup (170 g) of soup mixture into tuna. Divide mixture evenly among tortillas and roll up. Stir tomatoes into remaining soup mixture and spoon over top of each rollup. Place rollup seam side down in greased baking dish. Bake covered at 350°F (180°C, or gas mark 4) for 35 to 40 minutes. Top center of each tortilla with remaining cheese. Return to oven and bake 5 minutes, uncovered.

—

3 servings

Each with: 398 Calories (22% from Fat, 34% from Protein, 44% from Carb); 34 g Protein; 10 g Total Fat; 4 g Unsaturated Fat; 3 g Monounsaturated Fat; 2 g Polyunsaturated Fat; 44 g Carb; 5 g Fiber; 5 g Sugar; 529 mg Phosphorus; 314 mg Calcium; 890 mg Sodium; 1055 mg Potassium; 1178 IU Vitamin A; 41 mg ATE Vitamin E; 93 mg Vitamin C; 39 mg Cholesterol

Broccoli Fish Bake

A crispy bread crumb topping and a nice assortment of spices help make this fish and vegetable bake special. But it also provides lots of nutrition for not many calories.

1 cup (230 g) fat-free sour cream

1 cup (225 g) low fat mayonnaise

1 tablespoon (5 g) dried onion

2 teaspoons lemon pepper

¼ teaspoon white pepper

1 tablespoon (6 g) celery flakes

1 tablespoon (1 g) dried parsley

2 teaspoons lemon juice

⅛ teaspoon black pepper

20 ounces (570 g) broccoli

2 tablespoons (28 ml) lemon juice, divided

6 catfish fillets

¼ cup (30 g) bread crumbs

Mix first 9 ingredients and set aside. Spread broccoli in shallow casserole dish and drizzle with 1 tablespoon (15 ml) lemon juice. Layer fillets on broccoli and then spread the sour cream mixture. Top with sprinkled bread crumbs and remaining lemon juice. Bake covered at 350°F (180°C, or gas mark 4) for 45 minutes and then uncovered an additional 15 minutes until brown.

6 servings

Each with: 372 Calories (47% from Fat, 33% from Protein, 20% from Carb); 29 g Protein; 19 g Total Fat; 6 g Unsaturated Fat; 7 g Monounsaturated Fat; 3 g Polyunsaturated Fat; 18 g Carb; 4 g Fiber; 5 g Sugar; 444 mg Phosphorus; 119 mg Calcium; 486 mg Sodium; 885 mg Potassium; 921 IU Vitamin A; 64 mg ATE Vitamin E; 89 mg Vitamin C; 95 mg Cholesterol

Tuna Noodle (And Broccoli) Bake

Here's an updated version of the old familiar tuna noodle casserole. This one contains lots more vegetables and as a result lots more nutrition and fewer calories.

½ cup (80 g) onion, chopped

2 tablespoons (28 ml) olive oil

3 tablespoons (24 g) all purpose flour

2 cups (475 ml) skim milk

½ teaspoon savory

⅛ teaspoon black pepper

13 ounces (365 g) tuna, drained

10 ounces (280 g) broccoli, thawed

1 cup (110 g) Swiss cheese, shredded

8 ounces (225 g) egg noodles, cooked and drained

Cook onion in oil until tender; blend in flour. Add skim milk, savory, and black pepper. Cook until mixture boils and thickens. Combine all ingredients into 2-quart (1.9 L) casserole and bake uncovered at 350°F (180°C, or gas mark 4) for 30 minutes or until bubbly.

6 servings

Each with: 415 Calories (31% from Fat, 30% from Protein, 38% from Carb); 31 g Protein; 14 g Total Fat; 5 g Unsaturated Fat; 6 g Monounsaturated Fat; 2 g Polyunsaturated Fat; 40 g Carb; 3 g Fiber; 2 g Sugar; 478 mg Phosphorus; 375 mg Calcium; 106 mg Sodium; 581 mg Potassium; 696 IU Vitamin A; 107 mg ATE Vitamin E; 44 mg Vitamin C; 84 mg Cholesterol

Salmon with Mediterranean Relish

A tomato and olive relish gives this cold water fish a warm water feel, reminiscent of Greece or the Mediterranean islands. Salmon is very high in omega-3 fatty acids, and the vegetables take care of other nutrition. Microwaving the rice and asparagus makes preparation even easier.

½ teaspoon black pepper, or to taste

1 pound (455 g) salmon fillets

2 teaspoons ground cumin

2 cups (190 g) instant brown rice, uncooked

2¼ cups (535 ml) water

½ pound (225 g) asparagus

2 cups (360 g) tomatoes, diced

¼ cup (25 g) green olives, chopped

2 tablespoons (6 g) fresh basil, chopped

Preheat oven to 425°F (220°C, or gas mark 7). Coat a large baking sheet with nonstick vegetable oil spray. Sprinkle black pepper on both sides of salmon fillets. Rub cumin (½ teaspoon per fillet) into flesh-side of salmon. Place salmon skin-side down on prepared baking sheet. Roast 10 minutes until fillets are fork-tender. Meanwhile, combine brown rice and 2¼ cups (535 ml) water in a microwave-safe bowl with a lid. Cover and microwave on high for 5 minutes. Let stand 5 minutes. Fluff with a fork. Place the asparagus in a microwave-safe dish with a lid. Cover and microwave on high for 3 minutes until crisp-tender. To make the relish, combine tomatoes, olives, and basil in a medium bowl. Toss to combine. Serve the salmon with the relish spooned over top and the rice and asparagus on the side.

—

4 servings

Each with: 360 Calories (36% from Fat, 30% from Protein, 34% from Carb); 27 g Protein; 15 g Total Fat; 3 g Unsaturated Fat; 6 g Monounsaturated Fat; 5 g Polyunsaturated Fat; 30 g Carb; 5 g Fiber; 1 g Sugar; 398 mg Phosphorus; 81 mg Calcium; 151 mg Sodium; 825 mg Potassium; 1095 IU Vitamin A; 17 mg ATE Vitamin E; 28 mg Vitamin C; 67 mg Cholesterol

Spice It Up, Fill You Up Catfish Creole

This is actually a very simple, Creole-style recipe. Any white fish can be substituted for the catfish.

2 tablespoons (28 g) unsalted butter

1½ cups (240 g) onion, chopped

1 cup (100 g) celery, chopped

1 cup (150 g) green bell pepper, chopped

½ teaspoon garlic, minced

2 cups (360 g) no-salt-added tomatoes

1 lemon, sliced

1 tablespoon (15 ml) Worcestershire sauce

1 tablespoon (7 g) paprika

1 bay leaf

¼ teaspoon dried thyme

¼ teaspoon Tabasco sauce

2 pounds (900 g) catfish fillets

1½ cups (293 g) brown rice, cooked

2 pounds (900 g) cauliflower florets, steamed until crisp-tender

Melt the butter in a large skillet over medium heat. Add the onion, celery, green bell pepper, and garlic. Cook until soft. Add tomatoes and their liquid. Break the tomatoes with a spoon. Add lemon slices, Worcestershire sauce, paprika, bay leaf, thyme, and Tabasco sauce. Cook, stirring occasionally, for about 15 minutes or until the sauce is slightly thickened. Press fish pieces down into sauce and spoon some of the sauce over the top of the fish. Cover the pan and simmer gently until the fish flakes when prodded with a fork. Remove bay leaf. Serve over hot cooked rice with steamed cauliflower.

—
6 servings

Each with: 360 Calories (25% from Fat, 18% from Protein, 57% from Carb); 17 g Protein; 10 g Total Fat; 4 g Saturated Fat; 3 g Monounsaturated Fat; 2 g Polyunsaturated Fat; 53 g Carb; 9 g Fiber; 8 g Sugar; 355 mg Phosphorus; 90 mg Calcium; 107 mg Sodium; 874 mg Potassium; 1066 IU Vitamin A; 40 mg ATE Vitamin E; 112 mg Vitamin C; 35 mg Cholesterol

Quick Tuna Gumbo

Low in fat and high in taste and nutrition, this gumbo goes together quickly.

2 cups (390 g) brown rice, cooked

13 ounces (370 g) tuna, in water

10 ounces (280 g) okra, cut

2 cups (510 g) no-salt-added stewed tomatoes

8 ounces (225 g) no-salt-added tomato paste

4 ounces (115 g) green chilies, diced

1 cup (160 g) onion, cut fine

1 cup (235 ml) water

Cook rice according to package directions. Mix all other ingredients. Cook in a large sauce pan until okra is done. Serve over rice.

—
4 servings

Each with: 351 Calories (11% from Fat, 33% from Protein, 56% from Carb); 30 g Protein; 4 g Total Fat; 1 g Unsaturated Fat; 1 g Monounsaturated Fat; 2 g Polyunsaturated Fat; 51 g Carb; 9 g Fiber; 14 g Sugar; 412 mg Phosphorus; 164 mg Calcium; 509 mg Sodium; 1404 mg Potassium; 1406 IU Vitamin A; 6 mg ATE Vitamin E; 50 mg Vitamin C; 40 mg Cholesterol

Salmon and Vegetables Teriyaki

This recipe gives you so much great tasting salmon and vegetables that you won't even think about the fact that dishes like this are usually made much less healthy by putting them over white rice.

¼ cup (60 ml) low sodium soy sauce

¼ cup (60 ml) rice wine vinegar

¼ cup (6 g) sugar substitute, such as Splenda

¼ teaspoon garlic powder

½ teaspoon ground ginger

¼ teaspoon black pepper

1 pound (455 g) salmon fillets, cubed

2 cups (240 g) zucchini, sliced

1½ cups (240 g) onion, quartered

1½ cups (225 g) red bell pepper, cubed

2 cups (200 g) cauliflower florets

1 pound (455 g) mushrooms, sliced in half

2 tablespoons (28 ml) oil

2 tablespoons (16 g) cornstarch

Combine soy sauce, vinegar, sugar substitute, and spices. Stir until sugar is dissolved. Place fish in one plastic zipper bag and vegetables in another. Divide sauce between the 2 bags. Seal and marinate in refrigerator at least one hour, turning occasionally. Drain, reserving sauce. Heat oil in wok. Add vegetables and stir-fry 5 minutes. Add fish and stir-fry one more minute. Stir cornstarch into reserved marinade, add to wok, and cook and stir until thickened.

—
4 servings

Each with: 375 Calories (47% from Fat, 30% from Protein, 23% from Carb); 29 g Protein; 20 g Total Fat; 4 g Saturated Fat; 6 g Monounsaturated Fat; 9 g Polyunsaturated Fat; 23 g Carb; 6 g Fiber; 10 g Sugar; 438 mg Phosphorus; 55 mg Calcium; 91 mg Sodium; 1241 mg Potassium; 1939 IU Vitamin A; 17 mg ATE Vitamin E; 155 mg Vitamin C; 67 mg Cholesterol

Sweet Spicy Fish

This salmon is a real taste treat as well as being at the top of the nutritional ladder. Teamed with brown rice and steamed veggies, it makes a great meal.

1½ pounds (680 g) salmon fillets, cut ¾-inch (1.9 cm) thick

¼ cup (85 g) honey

¼ cup (60 ml) low sodium soy sauce

2 tablespoons (28 ml) lemon juice

1 tablespoon (15 ml) sesame oil

¼ teaspoon red pepper flakes

½ teaspoon black pepper

3 cups (585 g) brown rice, cooked

3 cups (257 g) broccoli and cauliflower mix, steamed until crisp-tender

Place fish in glass or ceramic baking dish. Combine honey, soy, lemon juice, sesame oil, red pepper flakes, and black pepper and pour over fish to coat. Cover with plastic wrap and marinate 30 minutes before cooking. Light barbecue grill. When coals are ready, oil grill with cooking spray and put in place. Place fish on grill, skin side down. Cover and co k 5 minutes. Drizzle fish with marinade and cook 3 minutes more or until fish turns opaque. Serve with cooked rice and steamed vegetables.

—
6 servings

Each with: 401 Calories (35% from Fat, 27% from Protein, 38% from Carb); 27 g Protein; 16 g Total Fat; 3 g Unsaturated Fat; 6 g Monounsaturated Fat; 6 g Polyunsaturated Fat; 38 g Carb; 3 g Fiber; 13 g Sugar; 387 mg Phosphorus; 48 mg Calcium; 441 mg Sodium; 628 mg Potassium; 379 IU Vitamin A; 17 mg ATE Vitamin E; 46 mg Vitamin C; 67 mg Cholesterol

Teriyaki Fish with Rice and Broccoli

This is an Teriyaki flavored catfish dish. For those of you (like me) who love Chinese food, it doesn't get any better than this.

¼ cup (31 g) all purpose flour

⅛ teaspoon black pepper

12 ounces (340 g) catfish fillets, cut in 1-inch (2.5 cm) cubes

2 tablespoons (28 ml) olive oil

¼ cup (60 ml) low sodium soy sauce

¼ cup (6 g) sugar substitute, such as Splenda

½ teaspoon sesame oil

¼ cup (12 g) chives, chopped

6 cups (426 g) broccoli florets, steamed until crisp-tender

3 cups (585 g) brown rice, cooked

Combine the flour and black pepper in a zipper bag. Add the fish and shake to coat. Heat the oil in a large skillet. Add the fish and cook until done. Remove from skillet. Add the soy sauce and sugar substitute to the pan. Cook and stir until the sugar substitute is melted. Stir in the sesame oil. Add the fish and chives and stir to coat. Serve with broccoli over rice.

—
4 servings

Each with: 426 Calories (33% from Fat, 20% from Protein, 47% from Carb); 22 g Protein; 16 g Total Fat; 3 g Saturated Fat; 9 g Monounsaturated Fat; 3 g Polyunsaturated Fat; 51 g Carb; 6 g Fiber; 3 g Sugar; 399 mg Phosphorus; 91 mg Calcium; 622 mg Sodium; 834 mg Potassium; 1045 IU Vitamin A; 13 mg ATE Vitamin E; 120 mg Vitamin C; 40 mg Cholesterol

Salmon and Pasta Caesar Salad

Perfect for a summer lunch or dinner, this tasty salad full of good things will be a real pleaser. And it will please you even more when you noticed that it only contains about 350 calories per serving.

8 ounces (225 g) whole wheat pasta

16 ounces (455 g) canned salmon, broken into pieces

¼ cup (30 g) zucchini, thinly sliced

¼ cup (25 g) celery, thinly sliced

¼ cup (48 g) pimento

¼ cup (60 ml) olive oil

1 tablespoon (15 ml) white wine vinegar

½ teaspoon Dijon mustard

½ teaspoon lemon juice

⅛ teaspoon garlic powder

lettuce leaves

Cook pasta according to package directions. Cool. In bowl, combine the next four ingredients. In blender container, combine the next four ingredients. Blend until smooth. Pour over salad ingredients. Cover and chill several hours. To serve, line salad plates with lettuce. Spoon salad onto leaves.

—

4 servings

Each with: 356 Calories (51% from Fat, 31% from Protein, 18% from Carb); 28 g Protein; 20 g Total Fat; 4 g Unsaturated Fat; 12 g Monounsaturated Fat; 3 g Polyunsaturated Fat; 16 g Carb; 2 g Fiber; 1 g Sugar; 460 mg Phosphorus; 297 mg Calcium; 103 mg Sodium; 427 mg Potassium; 440 IU Vitamin A; 20 mg ATE Vitamin E; 12 mg Vitamin C; 44 mg Cholesterol

Fish Mexicali

With the flavor of salsa and loaded with healthy red and yellow bell peppers, this Mexican casserole is sure to please.

1½ cups (143 g) instant brown rice

16 ounces (455 g) salsa

1 teaspoon dried thyme

1 cup (150 g) red bell pepper, sliced

1 cup (150 g) yellow bell pepper, sliced

1½ pounds (680 g) catfish fillets

¼ teaspoon black pepper

½ teaspoon paprika

4 tablespoons (4 g) fresh cilantro

In a microwaveable casserole dish, stir rice, salsa, and thyme. Cover and microwave on high for 7 minutes, stirring once or twice. Stir in red bell pepper. Place fish fillets on top of rice. Sprinkle with black pepper and paprika. Cover and microwave on high 4 or 5 minutes. Let stand 5 minutes. Garnish with cilantro.

—

4 servings

Each with: 367 Calories (35% from Fat, 33% from Protein, 32% from Carb); 31 g Protein; 14 g Total Fat; 3 g Unsaturated Fat; 6 g Monounsaturated Fat; 3 g Polyunsaturated Fat; 30 g Carb; 5 g Fiber; 7 g Sugar; 458 mg Phosphorus; 72 mg Calcium; 589 mg Sodium; 983 mg Potassium; 2448 IU Vitamin A; 26 mg ATE Vitamin E; 175 mg Vitamin C; 80 mg Cholesterol

Tuscan Shrimp with White Beans

This is one of those recipes that sounds a bit strange, with the mixture of shrimp and beans. But the first time we had it, it became an instant hit. Veggies and beans and low calorie shrimp make it lean but full of fiber and nutrients.

3 cups (786 g) cannellini beans

4 tablespoons (60 ml) olive oil

¾ pound (340 g) shrimp, peeled

1 teaspoon garlic, minced

½ cup (75 g) green bell pepper, diced

2 cups (360 g) no-salt-added tomatoes, diced

10 basil leaves

2 tablespoons (28 ml) lemon juice

2 tablespoons (8 g) fresh parsley

Drain the beans over a bowl and reserve the liquid. Put the white beans in a large skillet with just enough of their liquid to cover them. Add 2 tablespoons (28 ml) of the olive oil and bring the beans to a low simmer. Keep warm while you prepare the shrimp. Heat remaining oil in a large skillet over high heat. Add the shrimp and cook for about 1 minute, tossing frequently. Remove the shrimp with tongs to a bowl. Add the garlic to the pan and sauté until the garlic browns. Add the green bell pepper and cook for 1 minute. Add the tomato and basil and stir briefly and then add the lemon juice. Cook for about 1 minute and then stir in the shrimp. Toss well and cook briefly to reheat the shrimp. Spoon the white beans on a platter or individual plates. Top with the shrimp. Sprinkle with parsley.

—
4 servings

Each with: 434 Calories (33% from Fat, 28% from Protein, 40% from Carb); 31 g Protein; 16 g Total Fat; 2 g Unsaturated Fat; 10 g Monounsaturated Fat; 2 g Polyunsaturated Fat; 44 g Carb; 10 g Fiber; 4 g Sugar; 419 mg Phosphorus; 184 mg Calcium; 141 mg Sodium; 993 mg Potassium; 607 IU Vitamin A; 46 mg ATE Vitamin E; 41 mg Vitamin C; 129 mg Cholesterol

Greek Shrimp Bake

Feta cheese and ripe olives give this baked shrimp dish the flavor of Greece. Lots of veggies make it nutritious.

1 cup (190 g) brown rice, uncooked

2 cups (475 g) low sodium chicken broth

1 cup (100 g) celery, sliced

½ cup (80 g) onion, chopped

2 tablespoons (28 ml) olive oil

16 ounces (455 g) no-salt-added stewed tomatoes

1½ pounds (680 g) shrimp, shelled

¾ cup (113 g) feta cheese, crumbled

½ cup (70 g) ripe olives, sliced

1 teaspoon dill weed

Prepare rice according to package directions using chicken broth in place of the water. In a large pan, cook celery and onion in oil until tender. Add tomatoes, stir in rice, ½ of shrimp, cheese, ½ of olives, and dill weed. Turn into 2-quart (1.9 L) casserole. Top with rest of shrimp. Bake uncovered at 350°F (180°C, or gas mark 4) for 25 minutes. Garnish with the rest of the olives.

—
6 servings

Each with: 378 Calories (31% from Fat, 33% from Protein, 36% from Carb); 31 g Protein; 13 g Total Fat; 4 g Unsaturated Fat; 6 g Monounsaturated Fat; 2 g Polyunsaturated Fat; 34 g Carb; 3 g Fiber; 5 g Sugar; 446 mg Phosphorus; 211 mg Calcium; 685 mg Sodium; 593 mg Potassium; 560 IU Vitamin A; 85 mg ATE Vitamin E; 10 mg Vitamin C; 189 mg Cholesterol

Shrimp Pasta Primavera

The lemon juice gives this a distinctive flavor while complementing the shrimp nicely. It contains a healthy amount of vegetables (in both senses of the phrase), while still staying within our diet, so why not enjoy it?

8 ounces (225 g) whole wheat fettuccine

1 tablespoon (15 ml) olive oil

2 cups (142 g) broccoli florets

4 ounces (115 g) fresh green beans

½ cup (75 g) red bell pepper, cut in strips

1 pound (455 g) shrimp, peeled and deveined

¼ cup (60 ml) lemon juice

½ cup (120 ml) low sodium chicken broth

1 tablespoon (1.5 g) sugar substitute, such as Splenda

1 tablespoon (8 g) cornstarch

Cook fettuccini according to package directions and drain. Heat oil in a large skillet. Add vegetables and cook for 3 to 4 minutes, stirring frequently. Stir in shrimp and continue to cook for 4 more minutes. In a small bowl, combine remaining ingredients. Stir into shrimp mixture. Cook 1 to 2 minutes longer until thickened and bubbly. Stir in cooked fettuccini and cook until heated through.

—
4 servings

Each with: 384 Calories (14% from Fat, 34% from Protein, 52% from Carb); 33 g Protein; 6 g Total Fat; 1 g Saturated Fat; 3 g Monounsaturated Fat; 2 g Polyunsaturated Fat; 52 g Carb; 1 g Fiber; 1 g Sugar; 422 mg Phosphorus; 117 mg Calcium; 255 mg Sodium; 567 mg Potassium; 2013 IU Vitamin A; 61 mg ATE Vitamin E; 79 mg Vitamin C; 172 mg Cholesterol

Seafood Alfredo That You Can Eat

Generally when we think of Alfredo, we think of a dish loaded with fat because of oil, butter, cream, and cheese. But it doesn't have to be so. Our version is still creamy and gets its flavor from generous amounts of seafood, salmon, and vegetables. So you can eat it and still stay on your diet.

8 ounces (225 g) shrimp

8 ounces (225 g) scallops

½ pound (225 g) salmon fillets, cubed

1 teaspoon garlic, chopped

3 tablespoons (45 ml) olive oil

1 cup (160 g) onion, cut in wedges

1 cup (150 g) red bell pepper, sliced

1 cup (71 g) broccoli florets

3 tablespoons (24 g) all purpose flour

1½ cups (355 ml) skim milk

1 teaspoon Italian seasoning

¼ cup (25 g) Parmesan cheese

8 ounces (225 g) whole wheat spaghetti, cooked according to package directions

In a large saucepan, sauté shrimp, scallops, salmon, and garlic in 2 tablespoons (28 ml) olive oil until just cooked through. Remove and sauté vegetables in remaining oil. Shake together flour and skim milk. Add to pan along with Italian seasoning. Cook and stir until thickened and just beginning to boil. Stir in cheese. Serve over pasta.

—
6 servings

Each with: 402 Calories (29% from Fat, 31% from Protein, 40% from Carb); 32 g Protein; 13 g Total Fat; 3 g Saturated Fat; 7 g Monounsaturated Fat; 3 g Polyunsaturated Fat; 41 g Carb; 4 g Fiber; 2 g Sugar; 435 mg Phosphorus; 194 mg Calcium; 273 mg Sodium; 647 mg Potassium; 1408 IU Vitamin A; 79 mg ATE Vitamin E; 64 mg Vitamin C; 111 mg Cholesterol

Crawfish Pie

Or you can call it crayfish if you prefer (and aren't from Louisiana). This relatively uncommon seafood livens up this pie, which is also filled with lots of healthy veggies.

¾ cup (113 g) red bell pepper, chopped

1 cup (160 g) onion, chopped

½ cup (50 g) celery, chopped

2 tablespoons (28 g) unsalted butter

1½ pounds (680 g) crawfish tails

½ cup (50 g) green onion, chopped

½ cup (30 g) fresh parsley, minced

½ teaspoon black pepper

⅛ teaspoon cayenne pepper papper

½ teaspoon garlic powder

2 pie crusts

Sauté red bell pepper, onion, and celery in butter until tender. Add crawfish tails, green onion, parsley, and seasonings. Place half of the pie crust dough in a 9-inch (23 cm) pie pan. Fill with the cooled filling. Place top crust on pie, moisten edges, and seal edges. Cut two or three 1-inch long (2.5 cm) slits in the top crust. Bake for 10 minutes at 450°F (230°C, or gas mark 8); lower oven to 375°F (190°C, or gas mark 5) and cook for 35 minutes longer or until crust is golden brown.

—
6 servings

Each with: 442 Calories (51% from Fat, 19% from Protein, 30% from Carb); 21 g Protein; 25 g Total Fat; 8 g Unsaturated Fat; 10 g Monounsaturated Fat; 6 g Polyunsaturated Fat; 33 g Carb; 4 g Fiber; 3 g Sugar; 309 mg Phosphorus; 60 mg Calcium; 396 mg Sodium; 495 mg Potassium; 1324 IU Vitamin A; 49 mg ATE Vitamin E; 46 mg Vitamin C; 132 mg Cholesterol

Oven Fish Chowder

This delicious and nutritious fish chowder bakes in the oven while you do other things.

1 pound (455 g) haddock

2 potatoes, peeled and cubed

1 cup (160 g) onion, chopped

½ teaspoon garlic, sliced

¼ teaspoon dill weed

½ cup (120 ml) dry white wine

½ cup (120 ml) boiling water

1 bay leaf

½ cup (61 g) carrot, sliced

1 tablespoon (14 g) unsalted butter, in chunks

⅛ teaspoon black pepper

14 ounces (425 ml) fat-free evaporated milk

Put all ingredients, except evaporated milk, into large casserole. Cover and bake at 375°F (190°C, or gas mark 5) for 1 hour. Heat evaporated milk to scalding and add to chowder. Stir to break up fish or cut up with knife.

—
4 servings

Each with: 391 Calories (10% from Fat, 36% from Protein, 53% from Carb); 33 g Protein; 4 g Total Fat; 2 g Unsaturated Fat; 1 g Monounsaturated Fat; 0 g Polyunsaturated Fat; 49 g Carb; 4 g Fiber; 14 g Sugar; 535 mg Phosphorus; 372 mg Calcium; 218 mg Sodium; 1641 mg Potassium; 2493 IU Vitamin A; 160 mg ATE Vitamin E; 24 mg Vitamin C; 76 mg Cholesterol

Quick and Easy Salmon Stew

This is an easy way to make stew using canned salmon. It can easily be put together when you get home from work and still have dinner on the table at a reasonable hour.

1 cup (122 g) carrot, sliced

1½ cups (240 g) onion, chopped

16 ounces (455 g) canned salmon

10 ounces (280 g) frozen corn

¼ teaspoon black pepper

14 ounces (425 ml) fat-free evaporated milk

3 cups (700 ml) skim milk

Cook carrots and onion until tender. In large pot, combine carrot, onion, salmon with juice, corn, black pepper, and evaporated milk. Add skim milk and bring to a boil, stirring constantly. Turn burner off and continue to stir until mixture stops boiling.

—

4 servings

Each with: 413 Calories (17% from Fat, 41% from Protein, 42% from Carb); 42 g Protein; 8 g Total Fat; 2 g Unsaturated Fat; 3 g Monounsaturated Fat; 2 g Polyunsaturated Fat; 44 g Carb; 4 g Fiber; 18 g Sugar; 892 mg Phosphorus; 860 mg Calcium; 343 mg Sodium; 1387 mg Potassium; 4688 IU Vitamin A; 250 mg ATE Vitamin E; 14 mg Vitamin C; 52 mg Cholesterol

Salmon and Peanut Butter Stew

This is vaguely Thai, with its ginger and peanut flavors, but really hard to define. Whatever you call it, it tastes good and is full of nutrition.

⅓ cup (53 g) onion, chopped

⅓ cup (33 g) celery, chopped

½ cup (75 g) red bell pepper, sliced

2½ tablespoons (35 g) butter

¼ teaspoon ground ginger

¼ teaspoon turmeric

½ teaspoon black pepper

14 ounces (390 g) no-salt-added tomatoes, chopped

⅔ cup (160 ml) water

½ pound (225 g) salmon steaks

¾ cup (195 g) peanut butter, chunky

3 cups (585 g) brown rice, cooked

1 teaspoon lemon juice

Sauté onion, celery, and red bell pepper in the butter. Add ginger, turmeric, black pepper, tomatoes, and water; bring to boil. Cover. Simmer for 20 minutes at medium heat. Season and broil salmon until done. Heat peanut butter until it's melted and add to mixture. Place salmon on bed of rice. Squeeze lemon juice on salmon and cover with stew and serve.

—

6 servings

Each with: 426 Calories (52% from Fat, 17% from Protein, 31% from Carb); 18 g Protein; 25 g Total Fat; 7 g Unsaturated Fat; 10 g Monounsaturated Fat; 6 g Polyunsaturated Fat; 34 g Carb; 4 g Fiber; 6 g Sugar; 246 mg Phosphorus; 53 mg Calcium; 76 mg Sodium; 618 mg Potassium; 681 IU Vitamin A; 45 mg ATE Vitamin E; 36 mg Vitamin C; 35 mg Cholesterol

Thick and Rich Fish Chowder

This makes great chowder, flavorful and filling.

2 tablespoons (28 ml) olive oil

2 cups (320 g) chopped onion

1 cup (70 g) mushrooms, sliced

1 cup (100 g) celery, chopped

5 cups (1.1 L) low sodium chicken broth, divided

4 medium potatoes, diced

2 pounds (900 g) cod, diced into ½-inch (1.3 cm) cubes

⅛ teaspoon seafood seasoning

¼ teaspoon black pepper

¼ cup (31 g) all purpose flour

3 cups (700 ml) fat-free evaporated milk

In a large stockpot, heat oil over medium heat. Sauté onion, mushrooms, and celery until tender. Add 4 cups (950 ml) chicken broth and potatoes; simmer for 10 minutes. Add fish and simmer another 10 minutes. Season to taste with seafood seasoning and black pepper. Mix together remaining broth and flour until smooth; stir into soup. Cook until slightly thickened. Remove from heat and stir in evaporated milk. Serve.

—

8 servings

Each with: 390 Calories (13% from Fat, 36% from Protein, 51% from Carb); 35 g Protein; 6 g Total Fat; 1 g Saturated Fat; 3 g Monounsaturated Fat; 1 g Polyunsaturated Fat; 50 g Carb; 4 g Fiber; 15 g Sugar; 601 mg Phosphorus; 337 mg Calcium; 241 mg Sodium; 1885 mg Potassium; 505 IU Vitamin A; 127 mg ATE Vitamin E; 42 mg Vitamin C; 53 mg Cholesterol

TIP:

You can substitute other fish or a combination of different types of fish for the cod.

Alaska Salmon Chowder

They know how to make hearty, warming, filling soups in Alaska. And this chowder is a prime example. But it's loaded with so much salmon and so many vegetables that you won't believe its low calorie count.

1 cup (160 g) onion, chopped

2 tablespoons (28 ml) olive oil

2 medium potatoes, diced

1 cup (122 g) carrot, sliced

20 ounces (570 g) frozen broccoli

2 cups (475 ml) low sodium chicken broth

32 ounces (900 g) salmon

14 ounces (425 g) fat-free evaporated milk

2 tablespoons (16 g) cornstarch

4 cups (950 ml) skim milk

Sauté chopped onion in olive oil in saucepan. Add vegetables and broth. Simmer until vegetables are tender. Add flaked salmon and evaporated milk mixed with cornstarch and heat. Add the 4 cups (950 ml) of skim milk just before serving and reheat.

—

8 servings

Each with: 408 Calories (24% from Fat, 38% from Protein, 39% from Carb); 38 g Protein; 11 g Total Fat; 3 g Unsaturated Fat; 5 g Monounsaturated Fat; 2 g Polyunsaturated Fat; 39 g Carb; 4 g Fiber; 8 g Sugar; 765 mg Phosphorus; 661 mg Calcium; 274 mg Sodium; 1495 mg Potassium; 2916 IU Vitamin A; 154 mg ATE Vitamin E; 77 mg Vitamin C; 49 mg Cholesterol

Dinners: Vegetarian

Vegetarian meals are another great choice for healthy, reduced calorie eating. They are naturally low in fats in general and saturated fats in particular. This makes it easy to achieve that high nutrient, low calorie balance that we are looking for. They also offer a tremendous variety of flavors, adding variety to your mega meal plan. We try to have at least one vegetarian dinner a week, and I often eat meatless lunches.

Meal in a Potato

You'll really get your veggies in this recipe. And you'll also get so much taste and volume that you won't even think about the fact that it is meatless.

1 pound (455 g) cauliflower florets, steamed until crisp-tender

1 pound (455 g) broccoli florets, steamed until crisp-tender

1 cup (160 g) onion, steamed until crisp-tender

1 cup (150 g) red bell pepper, steamed until crisp-tender

4 large potatoes, baked

1 cup (110 g) low fat Swiss cheese

Steam vegetables. Cook potatoes in oven or microwave until done. Split and top with hot vegetables. Sprinkle with cheese.

—
4 servings

Each with: 408 Calories (6% from Fat, 19% from Protein, 74% from Carb); 21 g Protein; 3 g Total Fat; 1 g Saturated Fat; 1 g Monounsaturated Fat; 1 g Polyunsaturated Fat; 80 g Carb; 13 g Fiber; 10 g Sugar; 451 mg Phosphorus; 424 mg Calcium; 157 mg Sodium; 1675 mg Potassium; 1988 IU Vitamin A; 13 mg ATE Vitamin E; 247 mg Vitamin C; 12 mg Cholesterol

A Little Different Stuffed Pepper

Peas and carrots, as well as finely chopped walnuts, give these stuffed peppers not only a nutritional boost, but a flavor boost as well.

4 green bell peppers

1 tablespoon (15 ml) olive oil

1 cup (160 g) onion, chopped

½ teaspoon garlic, minced

1 teaspoon dried oregano

1 teaspoon dried basil

½ cup (61 g) carrot, julienned

1 cup (150 g) peas, fresh or frozen

1 cup (180 g) tomato, diced

⅓ cup (40 g) walnuts, finely chopped

1½ cups (293 g) brown rice, cooked

2 cups (490 g) low sodium spaghetti sauce

Preheat oven to 350°F (180°C, or gas mark 4). Wash and clean green bell peppers. Cut off tops and remove seeds and membrane. Steam peppers 3 to 4 minutes. Meanwhile, heat oil in wok or large skillet and add onion and garlic. Sauté 1 minute. Add herbs, carrot, and peas. Continue to cook 3 to 5 minutes or until carrots are tender, stirring constantly. Reduce heat and add the tomato, walnuts, brown rice, and ½ cup (123 g) tomato sauce. Heat through. Stuff mixture into peppers. Spread ½ cup (123 g) sauce in bottom of baking dish. Stand peppers upright. Pour remaining sauce over the tops of peppers. Bake in oven for 30 minutes.

—
4 servings

Each with: 405 Calories (35% from Fat, 10% from Protein, 55% from Carb); 11 g Protein; 17 g Total Fat; 2 g Unsaturated Fat; 8 g Monounsaturated Fat; 5 g Polyunsaturated Fat; 58 g Carb; 12 g Fiber; 22 g Sugar; 248 mg Phosphorus; 99 mg Calcium; 186 mg Sodium; 1129 mg Potassium; 3861 IU Vitamin A; 0 mg ATE Vitamin E; 147 mg Vitamin C; 0 mg Cholesterol

Stuffed Tomatoes

Cheese, rice, and fresh herbs make the filling of these stuffed tomatoes tasty as well as nutritious. It's perfect for a summer meal when fresh tomatoes are plentiful.

10 large tomatoes

2 cups (390 g) brown rice, cooked

1 cup (160 g) onion, chopped

1 teaspoon garlic, minced

¼ cup (16 g) fresh dill

¼ cup (15 g) fresh parsley, chopped

¼ cup (65 g) no-salt-added tomato paste

¼ cup (60 ml) water

1 cup (115 g) low fat cheddar cheese

¼ cup (60 ml) olive oil

¼ teaspoon black pepper

Slice tops from tomatoes and scoop out centers. Discard the hard center. Place in baking pan. Mix all ingredients together and spoon into tomato cups. Replace tops. Pour in enough boiling water to cover bottom of pan. Cover and bake at 350°F (180°C, or gas mark 4) degrees for about 45 minutes and then uncover and bake until brown and done.

—
5 servings

Each with: 367 Calories (55% from Fat, 6% from Protein, 40% from Carb); 5 g Protein; 23 g Total Fat; 3 g Unsaturated Fat; 16 g Monounsaturated Fat; 3 g Polyunsaturated Fat; 38 g Carb; 6 g Fiber; 3 g Sugar; 154 mg Phosphorus; 41 mg Calcium; 44 mg Sodium; 926 mg Potassium; 2344 IU Vitamin A; 0 mg ATE Vitamin E; 87 mg Vitamin C; 0 mg Cholesterol

Savory Lentil Pie

This crustless pie has a crunchy topping from cracker crumbs, which are lower in calories and fat than pie crust. Lentils add fiber and protein and vegetables up the nutrition but not the calorie count. Nicely spicy, it's a great choice for a cool night.

⅔ cup (128 g) lentils, rinsed

2 cups (475 ml) water

1 cup (160 g) onion, chopped

1 cup (122 g) carrot, sliced

½ cup (50 g) celery, sliced

6 cups (1.4 L) low sodium vegetable broth

3 medium potatoes, cubed

½ teaspoon dried sage

½ teaspoon dried parsley

3 tablespoons (42 g) unsalted butter

3 tablespoons (24 g) all purpose flour

1 cup (100 g) cracker crumbs

Cook lentils in 2 cups (475 ml) of water on low heat. Cook onion, carrot, and celery in broth for 10 minutes. Add potatoes and cook vegetables 20 more minutes. Meanwhile, add sage and parsley to lentils. Prepare a thickening agent by melting butter in a skillet, adding flour, and then 1 cup (235 ml) of liquid from the cooking vegetables. Drain vegetables (keeping extra liquid for possible use if the filling is too thick). Mix everything in a baking dish, put cracker crumbs on top, and bake at 350°F (180°C, or gas mark 4) until brown.

—
6 servings

Each with: 435 Calories (26% from Fat, 10% from Protein, 64% from Carb); 11 g Protein; 13 g Total Fat; 5 g Unsaturated Fat; 4 g Monounsaturated Fat; 2 g Polyunsaturated Fat; 70 g Carb; 8 g Fiber; 4 g Sugar; 253 mg Phosphorus; 115 mg Calcium; 309 mg Sodium; 1174 mg Potassium; 2822 IU Vitamin A; 48 mg ATE Vitamin E; 27 mg Vitamin C; 15 mg Cholesterol

Stuffed Cabbage Fingers

Unlike more traditional stuffed cabbage, this vegetarian version is formed into small rolls with individual leaves and then cooked in a cheesy tomato sauce. Tofu adds protein and an assortment of vegetables add other nutrients to this tasty meal.

1 head cabbage

2 tablespoons (28 ml) olive oil

1 teaspoon garlic, minced

1 cup (122 g) carrot, sliced thin

½ pound (225 g) mushrooms, sliced

1 cup (160 g) onion, chopped

2 cups (390 g) brown rice, cooked

8 ounces (225 g) firm tofu, cubed

1 tablespoon (7 g) caraway seeds

⅛ teaspoon dried thyme

¼ teaspoon dried basil

¼ teaspoon dried oregano

¼ teaspoon black pepper

3 cups (735 g) no-salt-added tomato sauce

½ cup (50 g) Parmesan cheese, grated

Rinse cabbage. Fill a pot with enough water to cover cabbage. Bring water to a boil. Place whole cabbage in water and blanch for 3 minutes, turning occasionally. Remove from pot and separate leaves from cabbage carefully. Place cabbage back in water for 2 to 3 minutes, if necessary, to remove inner leaves easily. Set aside. Heat oil in a large skillet. Add garlic and sauté for 1 minute. Add carrot, mushrooms, and onion and stir-fry for 3 minutes. Add rice; stir to combine. Add tofu, caraway seeds, thyme, basil, oregano, and black pepper; stir gently. Turn off heat. Spread cabbage leaves out and place 2 tablespoons (28 g) rice mixture in center of each. Roll up and secure with toothpicks. Cover bottom of two heatproof 9 × 9-inch (23 × 23 cm) baking dishes with tomato sauce. Carefully place rolls in. Top with remaining sauce and cheese. Place baking dishes in a preheated 350°F (180°C, or gas mark 4) oven and bake for 30 minutes.

—

4 servings

Each with: 397 Calories (30% from Fat, 17% from Protein, 53% from Carb); 17 g Protein; 14 g Total Fat; 4 g Unsaturated Fat; 7 g Monounsaturated Fat; 2 g Polyunsaturated Fat; 54 g Carb; 10 g Fiber; 16 g Sugar; 378 mg Phosphorus; 271 mg Calcium; 275 mg Sodium; 1469 mg Potassium; 4711 IU Vitamin A; 15 mg ATE Vitamin E; 59 mg Vitamin C; 11 mg Cholesterol

Good for You Good Tasting Veggie Rice Dinner

About as simple as a meal can get, an assortment of vegetables are sautéed and served over brown rice, with cheese sprinkled over. But don't be too fast to write it off. This meal has great taste appeal as well as great nutrition, all while holding down the calories.

¾ cup (143 g) brown rice

1 cup (160 g) onion, chopped

1 teaspoon garlic, minced

2 tablespoons (28 ml) olive oil

1 cup (120 g) zucchini, chopped

1 cup (150 g) green bell pepper, chopped

½ teaspoon dried oregano

⅛ teaspoon black pepper

1 cup (180 g) tomatoes, chopped

16 ounces (455 g) kidney beans, drained

½ cup (58 g) low fat cheddar cheese, shredded

Cook rice as per package directions. Sauté chopped onion and minced garlic in oil. Add zucchini and green bell pepper and seasonings. Sauté until crispy tender. Add tomatoes and beans and heat through. Serve over rice with shredded cheese on top.

—
4 servings

Each with: 396 Calories (21% from Fat, 18% from Protein, 61% from Carb); 18 g Protein; 9 g Total Fat; 2 g Unsaturated Fat; 6 g Monounsaturated Fat; 1 g Polyunsaturated Fat; 62 g Carb; 14 g Fiber; 3 g Sugar; 370 mg Phosphorus; 177 mg Calcium; 116 mg Sodium; 873 mg Potassium; 482 IU Vitamin A; 10 mg ATE Vitamin E; 49 mg Vitamin C; 3 mg Cholesterol

Eggplant Zucchini Casserole

Called it baked spaghetti, vegetable lasagna, or whatever you want, this vegetarian dish is healthy, tasty, and filling. Spaghetti teams with vegetables, primarily eggplant and zucchini, in an Italian-style baked casserole.

1 medium eggplant, peeled and sliced

2 cups (240 g) zucchini, sliced

28 ounces (758 g) low sodium spaghetti sauce

½ cup (50 g) celery, chopped

1 cup (150 g) green bell pepper, chopped

8 ounces (225 g) part skim mozzarella, grated

8 ounces (225 g) whole wheat spaghetti, broken into 1-inch (2.5 cm) pieces

Layer ½ eggplant slices in greased 9 × 13-inch (23 × 33 cm) baking dish, then ½ zucchini, then ½ spaghetti, ½ celery, and green bell pepper. Sprinkle with ½ cheese and ½ spaghetti sauce. Repeat layers. Bake, covered, at 350°F (180°C, or gas mark 4) for 1½ hours.

—
6 servings

Each with: 403 Calories (28% from Fat, 18% from Protein, 54% from Carb); 19 g Protein; 13 g Total Fat; 5 g Unsaturated Fat; 6 g Monounsaturated Fat; 1 g Polyunsaturated Fat; 58 g Carb; 11 g Fiber; 19 g Sugar; 362 mg Phosphorus; 367 mg Calcium; 291 mg Sodium; 974 mg Potassium; 1234 IU Vitamin A; 47 mg ATE Vitamin E; 44 mg Vitamin C; 24 mg Cholesterol

Warm Bean and Pasta Toss

A sort of warm pasta salad, this dish features beans and vegetables tossed with pasta and heated but not cooked.

8 ounces (225 g) whole wheat pasta, such as penne

2 cups (524 g) white beans, rinsed and drained

40 cherry tomatoes, halved

1 cup (150 g) green bell pepper, chopped

2 tablespoons (28 ml) olive oil

½ cup (20 g) fresh basil, chopped

½ teaspoon garlic cloves, minced

¼ cup (25 g) Parmesan cheese, grated

Cook noodles, drain, and return to pot. Toss with next 6 ingredients and warm for 5 minutes. Top with Parmesan cheese.

TIP:

You could serve over lettuce if desired.

—
4 servings

Each with: 341 Calories (25% from Fat, 17% from Protein, 57% from Carb); 16 g Protein; 10 g Total Fat; 2 g Unsaturated Fat; 6 g Monounsaturated Fat; 1 g Polyunsaturated Fat; 52 g Carb; 12 g Fiber; 1 g Sugar; 267 mg Phosphorus; 244 mg Calcium; 102 mg Sodium; 958 mg Potassium; 1623 IU Vitamin A; 7 mg ATE Vitamin E; 66 mg Vitamin C; 6 mg Cholesterol

Vegetarian Skillet Meal

This is like a frittata, but it's cooked in a covered skillet on top of the stove. Cast iron works really well for this. This great combination of vegetables held together by egg makes a really nutritious meal.

2 tablespoons (28 ml) olive oil

1 teaspoon garlic, minced

1½ cups (240 g) onion, thinly sliced

½ cup (120 ml) low sodium vegetable broth

1 cup (150 g) green bell pepper, diced

2 medium potatoes, cubed

2 cups (360 g) tomatoes, diced

2 cups (240 g) zucchini, diced

½ teaspoon black pepper

1 cup (82 g) eggplant, unpeeled, diced

2 cups (475 ml) egg substitute

Heat olive oil in large skillet. Add garlic. Cook until golden. Discard garlic. Add onion to hot oil. Sauté until tender. Add broth or water, green bell pepper, potatoes, tomatoes, zucchini, black pepper, and eggplant. Mix well. Pour egg substitute over. Cover and cook over low heat until vegetables are tender and eggs are set, about 30 minutes.

—
4 servings

Each with: 388 Calories (28% from Fat, 22% from Protein, 50% from Carb); 22 g Protein; 12 g Total Fat; 2 g Unsaturated Fat; 7 g Monounsaturated Fat; 3 g Polyunsaturated Fat; 49 g Carb; 7 g Fiber; 6 g Sugar; 337 mg Phosphorus; 132 mg Calcium; 397 mg Sodium; 1781 mg Potassium; 1201 IU Vitamin A; 0 mg ATE Vitamin E; 84 mg Vitamin C; 1 mg Cholesterol

Veggie Burgers You Can Love

Ever long for a big juicy burger but worry about the number of calories and the amount of fat? Worry no more. These burgers are big and juicy and lean. Mushrooms add extra moisture to the protein rich tofu and oat base. So enjoy.

2 cups (320 g) onion, chopped

¾ pound (340 g) mushrooms, chopped

1 teaspoon garlic, crushed

2 pounds (900 g) tofu

3 cups (240 g) rolled oats

10 ounces (280 g) frozen spinach, thawed and drained

2 tablespoons (28 ml) low sodium soy sauce

4 tablespoons (60 ml) Worcestershire sauce

½ teaspoon black pepper

1 teaspoon paprika

1 teaspoon lemon juice

8 whole wheat rolls

2 cups (320 g) tomatoes, sliced

8 leaves romaine lettuce

8 dill pickle halves

Sauté onion, mushrooms, and garlic in a small amount of water until they are softened and water is absorbed. Mash tofu in a large bowl. Add oats, spinach (make sure all excess water is removed), seasonings, and lemon juice. Mix well. Stir in onion–mushroom mixture. Shape into patties and place on nonstick cookie sheet. Bake at 350°F (180°C, or gas mark 4) for 20 minutes; turn over and then cook an additional 10 minutes. Serve on rolls with lettuce and tomato and pickle on the side.

---

8 servings

Each with: 352 Calories (20% from Fat, 20% from Protein, 60% from Carb); 18 g Protein; 8 g Total Fat; 1 g Unsaturated Fat; 2 g Monounsaturated Fat; 3 g Polyunsaturated Fat; 55 g Carb; 8 g Fiber; 9 g Sugar; 365 mg Phosphorus; 148 mg Calcium; 904 mg Sodium; 995 mg Potassium; 4362 IU Vitamin A; 0 mg ATE Vitamin E; 40 mg Vitamin C; 0 mg Cholesterol

Vegetarian Stroganoff

I know it may sound weird, but trust me here. This dish is definitely a stroganoff in flavor, but an assortment of vegetables take the place of the meat, keeping the calories low and the nutrition high.

1 pound (455 g) whole wheat noodles

2 tablespoons (28 ml) olive oil

2 cups (300 g) green bell pepper, diced

2½ cups (400 g) tomatoes, cut into wedges

2 cups (240 g) zucchini, diced

1 cup (82 g) eggplant, diced

1 cup (100 g) celery, diced

1 cup (100 g) green beans

¼ teaspoon black pepper

½ teaspoon ground cumin

1 tablespoon (10 g) chopped onion

1 teaspoon chili powder

2 tablespoons (3 g) fresh parsley, chopped

3 cups (690 g) fat-free sour cream

Boil the noodles. In the meantime, sauté the next 7 ingredients. When vegetables are translucent, add the next 4 ingredients and sauté a few minutes longer. As soon as the eggplant is cooked, add the last 2 ingredients as well as noodles that have been boiled and drained.

—
8 servings

Each with: 383 Calories (34% from Fat, 12% from Protein, 53% from Carb); 13 g Protein; 15 g Total Fat; 7 g Unsaturated Fat; 6 g Monounsaturated Fat; 1 g Polyunsaturated Fat; 54 g Carb; 3 g Fiber; 2 g Sugar; 277 mg Phosphorus; 144 mg Calcium; 67 mg Sodium; 596 mg Potassium; 1166 IU Vitamin A; 91 mg ATE Vitamin E; 53 mg Vitamin C; 35 mg Cholesterol

Did I Say Tofu Quiche?

Yes, I did, for want of a better term. And it works well, the tofu blending into the eggs and mayonnaise until it's not even noticeable as a separate ingredient. But it supercharges the dish, giving it great nutrient value for very few calories.

12 ounces (340 g) firm tofu, drained

1 cup (122 g) carrot, sliced

2 cups (240 g) zucchini, sliced

6 ounces (170 g) water chestnuts, sliced

¼ cup (25 g) green onion, sliced

1 cup (225 g) low fat mayonnaise

1½ cups (355 ml) egg substitute

Drain tofu by wrapping in cheesecloth and setting a weight on top of it. (A couple of dinner plates work well.) Let sit approximately 20 minutes. Chop vegetables. Mash tofu in large bowl with pastry blender or potato masher. Stir in mayonnaise until blended. Stir in egg substitute until just mixed. Stir in vegetables. Grease 9-inch (23 cm) baking dish. Pour mixture into dish and bake 1 hour at 350°F (180°C, or gas mark 4).

—

3 servings

Each with: 360 Calories (27% from Fat, 31% from Protein, 43% from Carb); 25 g Protein; 10 g Total Fat; 2 g Unsaturated Fat; 2 g Monounsaturated Fat; 4 g Polyunsaturated Fat; 35 g Carb; 6 g Fiber; 14 g Sugar; 362 mg Phosphorus; 147 mg Calcium; 950 mg Sodium; 1384 mg Potassium; 5920 IU Vitamin A; 0 mg ATE Vitamin E; 20 mg Vitamin C; 10 mg Cholesterol

Black Bean and Zucchini Quesadilla

This may sound like an unusual combination, but the zucchini takes on the Mexican flavor and it all works very well together. It also provides great nutrition.

2 cups (240 g) zucchini, chopped

1 cup (172 g) black beans, rinsed and drained

1 tablespoon (15 ml) olive oil

1 tablespoon (7 g) ground cumin

4 whole wheat tortillas, 8-inch (20 cm)

½ cup (58 g) cheddar cheese, shredded

¼ cup (65 g) salsa

Sauté first 4 ingredients for 5 minutes. Place mixture on tortillas; sprinkle with cheese. Fold in half and heat in skillet until cheese melts and tortilla is toasted. Top with salsa.

—

4 servings

Each with: 386 Calories (28% from Fat, 19% from Protein, 53% from Carb); 19 g Protein; 12 g Total Fat; 5 g Unsaturated Fat; 6 g Monounsaturated Fat; 1 g Polyunsaturated Fat; 52 g Carb; 10 g Fiber; 3 g Sugar; 330 mg Phosphorus; 219 mg Calcium; 337 mg Sodium; 1001 mg Potassium; 417 IU Vitamin A; 43 mg ATE Vitamin E; 13 mg Vitamin C; 17 mg Cholesterol

Dinner in a Dish Artichoke Pie

Meatless meals don't have to be tasteless, not do they have to be something that leaves you feeling like you haven't had a full dinner. This Italian-style pie is loaded with vegetables to give you a full feeling that will last.

¾ cups (175 ml) egg substitute

3 ounces (85 g) fat-free
cream cheese, softened

¾ teaspoon garlic powder

1 tablespoon dried chives

¼ teaspoon black pepper

1½ cups (173 g) part skim
mozzarella, shredded

1 cup (150 g) ricotta cheese

½ cup (115 g) low fat mayonnaise

1 can (6 ounces, or 170 g)
artichoke hearts

8 ounces (225 g) mushrooms,
sliced

1 cup (240 g) garbanzo beans,
cooked

½ cup (70 g) black olives, sliced

2 ounces (55 g) pimento,
drained and diced

2 tablespoons (8 g) fresh
parsley, chopped

One 9-inch (23 cm) pie shell,
unbaked

⅓ cup (33 g) Parmesan cheese,
grated

In a mixing bowl, beat egg substitute. Stir in cream cheese, garlic powder, chives, and black pepper. Stir in 1 cup (115 g) mozzarella, ricotta, and mayonnaise. Quarter 2 artichoke hearts and set aside 6 pieces. Chop remaining artichoke hearts; fold into cheese mixture. Fold in mushrooms, garbanzo beans, olives, pimento, and parsley. Turn mixture into pie shell. Bake in a 350°F (180°C, or gas mark 4) oven for 30 minutes. Top with remaining ½ cup (60 g) mozzarella and the Parmesan cheese. Bake about 15 minutes more until set. Let stand for 10 minutes. Top with quartered artichokes.

—
6 servings

Each with: 405 Calories (52% from Fat, 17% from Protein, 30% from Carb); 18 g Protein; 24 g Total Fat; 8 g Saturated Fat; 7 g Monounsaturated Fat; 2 g Polyunsaturated Fat; 31 g Carb; 5 g Fiber; 5 g Sugar; 295 mg Phosphorus; 246 mg Calcium; 771 mg Sodium; 540 mg Potassium; 932 IU Vitamin A; 75 mg ATE Vitamin E; 15 mg Vitamin C; 33 mg Cholesterol

Tamale Pie

A tasty chili flavored cornmeal crust wraps around a bean based filling with lots of vegetables in this pie. The result is the kind of thing you can serve to anyone and not worry about it being diet food.

FILLING

¼ cup (38 g) green bell pepper, chopped

¼ cup (25 g) celery, chopped

½ cup (80 g) onion, chopped

1 tablespoon (15 ml) olive oil

2 teaspoons chili powder

1 teaspoon ground cumin

1 teaspoon garlic, minced

2 cups (512 g) kidney beans, drained

2 tablespoons (32 g) no-salt-added tomato paste

½ cup (70 g) ripe olives

½ cup (82 g) corn

CRUST

1½ cups (210 g) cornmeal

1 cup (235 ml) cold water

2 cups (475 ml) boiling water

½ teaspoon chili powder

⅓ cup (38 g) low fat cheddar cheese, grated

Sauté vegetables for filling. When onions become translucent, add spices and crushed garlic. Mash beans. Mix beans and tomato paste into vegetables. Add olives and corn. Set aside. Stir cornmeal into 1 cup (235 ml) cold water. Then stir cornmeal mixture into 2 cups (475 ml) boiling water. Add chili powder. Cook and stir until thick. Press ⅔ of the cornmeal mixture into the bottom and sides of an 8 × 8-inch (20 × 20 cm) pan. Pour the bean mixture into the crust. Top with remaining cornmeal mixture. Sprinkle with cheese and bake at 350°F (180°C, or gas mark 4) for 30 minutes.

—
4 servings

Each with: 410 Calories (16% from Fat, 16% from Protein, 68% from Carb); 17 g Protein; 8 g Total Fat; 1 g Unsaturated Fat; 4 g Monounsaturated Fat; 1 g Polyunsaturated Fat; 70 g Carb; 15 g Fiber; 3 g Sugar; 260 mg Phosphorus; 147 mg Calcium; 257 mg Sodium; 705 mg Potassium; 867 IU Vitamin A; 7 mg ATE Vitamin E; 15 mg Vitamin C; 2 mg Cholesterol

Veggie Burritos

With the flavor of traditional burritos, but not the calorie count, these burritos are a great choice for lunch or dinner. Filled with an assortment of vegetables, they will leave you satisfied both by the taste and the volume.

1 cup (160 g) onion, finely chopped

1 teaspoon garlic, minced

2 tablespoons (28 ml) olive oil

1 teaspoon dried oregano

1 cup (150 g) green bell pepper, chopped

1 cup (120 g) zucchini, chopped

1 cup (110 g) carrot, grated

4 ounces (115 g) green chilies, chopped

1 teaspoon ground cumin

6 whole wheat tortillas, 8-inch (20 cm)

2 cups (476 g) refried beans, see recipe in chapter 14

1½ cups (173 g) low fat cheddar cheese, grated

½ cup (130 g) salsa

¼ cup (60 g) fat-free sour cream

Sauté onion and garlic in hot oil in a frying pan with oregano. Add the green bell pepper, zucchini, carrot, and chili peppers. Sauté 5 minutes until tender but not overcooked. Remove from heat and add cumin. Microwave the tortillas for 10 to 15 seconds to soften them. Spread about 2 tablespoons (28 g) refried beans in center of tortilla, add about ½ cup (115 g) of vegetable mixture, and sprinkle with cheese. Fold up sides and then roll the rest of the tortilla. Place seam side down on a cookie sheet. Bake at 350°F (180°C, or gas mark 4) for about 10 minutes until golden brown. Serve with salsa and sour cream.

TIP:

If you like your Mexican food spicy, feel free to add more chilies. Each 4 ounce (115 g) can only adds 4 calories per serving.

—
6 servings

Each with: 366 Calories (30% from Fat, 19% from Protein, 51% from Carb); 18 g Protein; 13 g Total Fat; 4 g Unsaturated Fat; 7 g Monounsaturated Fat; 1 g Polyunsaturated Fat; 49 g Carb; 8 g Fiber; 4 g Sugar; 336 mg Phosphorus; 272 mg Calcium; 632 mg Sodium; 601 mg Potassium; 2991 IU Vitamin A; 30 mg ATE Vitamin E; 41 mg Vitamin C; 18 mg Cholesterol

Bean and Guacamole Burritos

This is a delicious vegetarian Mexican meal, high in fiber and nutrition and low in saturated fat.

1 cup (190 g) brown rice, uncooked

¼ cup (38 g) green bell pepper, diced

¼ cup (45 g) onion, diced

4 ounces (115 g) green chilies, diced

¾ cup (195 g) salsa, divided

½ cup (119 g) refried beans, see recipe in chapter 14

6 tablespoons (88 g) guacamole

1 cup (47 g) romaine lettuce, shredded

2 whole wheat tortillas, 8-inch (20 cm)

Cook rice according to package directions, adding green bell pepper, onion, green chilies, and ¼ cup (65 g) salsa. Stir together beans and ½ cup (65 g) salsa. Microwave for 1 to 2 minutes. Place warm bean mixture, guacamole, and lettuce on tortillas and roll up. Serve with rice on the side.

—

2 servings

Each with: 408 Calories (20% from Fat, 12% from Protein, 68% from Carb); 13 g Protein; 9 g Total Fat; 2 g Unsaturated Fat; 5 g Monounsaturated Fat; 2 g Polyunsaturated Fat; 73 g Carb; 12 g Fiber; 6 g Sugar; 249 mg Phosphorus; 157 mg Calcium; 886 mg Sodium; 843 mg Potassium; 2459 IU Vitamin A; 0 mg ATE Vitamin E; 62 mg Vitamin C; 5 mg Cholesterol

Better Than It Sounds Pasta with Tofu

OK, it sounds funny, but it works. Tofu is crumbled and stir-fried with vegetables and then added to pasta sauce to produce a meal that is incredibly nutritious, but it's also even lower in calories than most of the meals here.

8 ounces (225 g) whole wheat pasta

1 tablespoon (15 ml) olive oil

1 cup (160 g) onion, chopped

½ teaspoon garlic, minced

14 ounces (390 g) firm tofu

2 teaspoons dried basil

8 ounces (225 g) mushrooms, sliced

2 cups (240 g) zucchini, sliced

25 ounces (700 g) low sodium spaghetti sauce

Cook pasta according to package directions. Heat the oil in a pan and add the chopped onion and garlic. When they get golden in color, add an entire block of firm tofu. Don't chop it but crumble it finely instead. Add the basil. Turn the heat down and let the tofu cook with the onion and spices for about 5 minutes. Meanwhile, chop the mushrooms and slice the zucchini. Stir them into the tofu mixture. Cook until mushrooms and zucchini are softened. Add the tomato sauce. Stir well. Heat through. Serve over the pasta.

—

4 servings

Each with: 301 Calories (26% from Fat, 20% from Protein, 54% from Carb); 16 g Protein; 9 g Total Fat; 1 g Unsaturated Fat; 4 g Monounsaturated Fat; 3 g Polyunsaturated Fat; 43 g Carb; 7 g Fiber; 6 g Sugar; 290 mg Phosphorus; 112 mg Calcium; 845 mg Sodium; 1308 mg Potassium; 868 IU Vitamin A; 4 mg ATE Vitamin E; 31 mg Vitamin C; 0 mg Cholesterol

Pizza Salad, Now There's a Combination

If you have a taste for pizza but are trying to get your recommended vegetables in for the day, this salad topped pizza may be the solution you are looking for.

3 large tomatoes

8 ounces (225 g) fresh mozzarella, shredded

2 tablespoons (10 g) Parmesan cheese

1 pizza crust, unbaked

2 cups (94 g) romaine lettuce, shredded

1 cup (150 g) green bell pepper, thinly sliced

1 cup (160 g) red onion, thinly sliced

1 cup (120 g) zucchini, thinly sliced

1 cup (71 g) broccoli florets

¼ cup (35 g) ripe olives, sliced

2 tablespoons (28 ml) Reduced Fat Italian Dressing, see recipe in chapter 2

Preheat oven to 450°F (230°C, or gas mark 8). Core tomatoes; slice into ¼-inch (6 mm) thick slices and set aside. Sprinkle mozzarella and Parmesan cheeses evenly over pizza crust. Top with tomato slices, slightly overlapping. Bake about 8 minutes or until cheese melts. Meanwhile, in medium bowl, combine romaine, green bell pepper, and olives. Sprinkle with Italian dressing. Toss to coat. Remove pizza from oven. Top with romaine mixture. Cut into wedges. Serve immediately.

6 servings

Each with: 385 Calories (29% from Fat, 19% from Protein, 52% from Carb); 18 g Protein; 12 g Total Fat; 5 g Saturated Fat; 5 g Monounsaturated Fat; 2 g Polyunsaturated Fat; 51 g Carb; 2 g Fiber; 3 g Sugar; 242 mg Phosphorus; 351 mg Calcium; 961 mg Sodium; 423 mg Potassium; 2252 IU Vitamin A; 49 mg ATE Vitamin E; 60 mg Vitamin C; 26 mg Cholesterol

Italian Oven Meal in a Pot

This Italian vegetarian dish, halfway between a soup and a casserole, cooks in the oven while you do other things. The cheeses add richness, and the beans and veggies take care of the nutrition.

1 cup (120 g) zucchini, sliced

1½ cups (240 g) onion, sliced

2 cups (480 g) garbanzo beans

2 cups (360 g) no-salt-added tomatoes, chopped

8 ounces (225 g) whole wheat pasta, cooked according to package directions

1½ cups (355 ml) dry white wine

2 teaspoons garlic, minced

1 teaspoon dried basil

1 bay leaf

2 ounces (55 g) Monterey Jack cheese, shredded

2 ounces (55 g) Romano cheese, grated

Combine zucchini, onion, beans, tomatoes and their liquid, pasta, wine, garlic, basil, and bay leaf in 3-quart (2.8 L) baking dish. Cover and bake at 400°F (200°C, or gas mark 6) for 1 hour, stirring once halfway through. Remove bay leaf. Stir in cheeses and bake 10 minutes longer.

6 servings

Each with: 376 Calories (18% from Fat, 19% from Protein, 64% from Carb); 16 g Protein; 7 g Total Fat; 4 g Saturated Fat; 2 g Monounsaturated Fat; 1 g Polyunsaturated Fat; 56 g Carb; 8 g Fiber; 5 g Sugar; 327 mg Phosphorus; 257 mg Calcium; 421 mg Sodium; 583 mg Potassium; 289 IU Vitamin A; 27 mg ATE Vitamin E; 21 mg Vitamin C; 18 mg Cholesterol

Pasta with Mushroom and Sun-Dried Tomato Sauce

A quick and very flavorful mushroom sauce with sun-dried tomatoes makes this pasta special. You'll love the way it tastes and fills, even without any meat.

1 pound (455 g) mushrooms, sliced

½ teaspoon garlic, minced

1 cup (55 g) sun-dried tomatoes, chopped

½ cup (120 ml) dry white wine

½ cup (120 ml) low sodium vegetable broth

¼ cup (15 g) Italian parsley, chopped

10 ounces (280 g) whole wheat pasta

¼ cup (25 g) Parmesan cheese

Combine all ingredients except pasta and cheese in a large saucepan. Cover and simmer for 1 hour. Cook pasta according to package directions. Serve with sauce, sprinkled with cheese.

4 servings

Each with: 392 Calories (17% from Fat, 18% from Protein, 65% from Carb); 18 g Protein; 8 g Total Fat; 2 g Saturated Fat; 3 g Monounsaturated Fat; 1 g Polyunsaturated Fat; 66 g Carb; 9 g Fiber; 2 g Sugar; 377 mg Phosphorus; 126 mg Calcium; 329 mg Sodium; 1004 mg Potassium; 698 IU Vitamin A; 7 mg ATE Vitamin E; 36 mg Vitamin C; 6 mg Cholesterol

Three Greens Lasagna

Many lasagna recipes contain spinach. But not many contain the nutritional boost of three greens, spinach, kale, and arugula, like this one does. It's so good that even confirmed meat eaters will agree that vegetarian meals can be delicious and satisfying.

1 pound (455 g) lasagna noodles, preferably whole wheat

16 ounces (455 g) fat-free cottage cheese

1 teaspoon dried thyme

1 teaspoon dried basil

1 teaspoon dried oregano

2 teaspoons garlic, minced

28 ounces (785 ml) low sodium spaghetti sauce

5 cups (335 g) kale

5 cups (100 g) arugula

5 cups (150 g) spinach

1 cup (180 g) roasted red peppers, diced

¼ cup (25 g) Parmesan cheese, grated

Cook lasagna noodles according to package directions. Preheat oven to 375°F (190°C, or gas mark 5). Mix cottage cheese, thyme, basil, oregano, and garlic in a medium bowl. Spread 1 cup (245 g) pasta sauce on the bottom of a 13 × 9-inch (33 × 23 cm) baking dish. Add one layer of cooked lasagna noodles. Top lasagna with greens and roasted red peppers. Spread spoonfuls of the cheese mixture over vegetables. Repeat layers, finishing with pasta and sauce. Sprinkle grated Parmesan on top of the lasagna and bake uncovered for about 40 minutes or until bubbly around the edges. Let the lasagna stand 10 minutes to make cutting easier. Slice into 8 pieces and serve.

—

8 servings

Each with: 408 Calories (17% from Fat, 19% from Protein, 64% from Carb); 20 g Protein; 8 g Total Fat; 2 g Unsaturated Fat; 4 g Monounsaturated Fat; 1 g Polyunsaturated Fat; 67 g Carb; 6 g Fiber; 14 g Sugar; 180 mg Phosphorus; 209 mg Calcium; 349 mg Sodium; 909 mg Potassium; 9736 IU Vitamin A; 10 mg ATE Vitamin E; 104 mg Vitamin C; 5 mg Cholesterol

Stuffed Shells Florentine

This is a vegetarian Italian meal that is low in fat, but high in nutrition, with the addition of extra vegetables to the mixture used to stuff the shells.

10 ounces (280 g) jumbo
pasta shells

1 cup (70 g) mushrooms,
chopped

1 cup (160 g) onion, chopped

1 cup (150 g) green bell
pepper, chopped

½ teaspoon garlic, minced

½ teaspoon onion powder

½ teaspoon dried parsley

¼ teaspoon black pepper

16 ounces (455 g) low fat
cottage cheese

20 ounces (570 g) frozen
spinach, thawed and
well drained

½ cup (120 ml) egg substitute

15 ounces (425 g) low sodium
marinara sauce

Preheat oven to 350°F (180°C, or gas mark 4). Cook pasta according to package instructions. Sauté mushrooms, onion, green bell pepper, garlic, and seasonings in a skillet sprayed with nonstick vegetable oil spray. Remove from heat and stir in cottage cheese, spinach, and egg substitute. Spoon the mix into the shells. Spread ½ cup (123 g) of the sauce into the bottom of a 13 × 9-inch (33 × 23 cm) baking dish and place the shells in the dish. Top with the rest of the sauce and bake 35 to 40 minutes.

—
5 servings

Each with: 412 Calories (14% from Fat, 27% from Protein, 59% from Carb); 28 g Protein; 6 g Total Fat; 2 g Unsaturated Fat; 2 g Monounsaturated Fat; 2 g Polyunsaturated Fat; 61 g Carb; 6 g Fiber; 3 g Sugar; 358 mg Phosphorus; 227 mg Calcium; 828 mg Sodium; 1218 mg Potassium; 11 212 IU Vitamin A; 19 mg ATE Vitamin E; 65 mg Vitamin C; 8 mg Cholesterol

Eggplant Lasagna

Eggplant takes the place of noodles in this vegetarian lasagna, providing increased nutrition and decreased calories. But the flavor is still great and a generous helping will fill you up and keep you that way.

½ pound (225 g) plum tomatoes, halved and seeded

½ teaspoon garlic, minced

4 tablespoons (60 ml) olive oil

1 teaspoon black pepper, divided

3 pounds (1⅓ kg) eggplant, sliced lengthwise ¼-inch (6 mm) thick

1 cup (250 g) ricotta

¼ cup (60 ml) egg substitute

½ cup (20 g) fresh basil, chopped

¼ cup (25 g) Parmesan, grated

4 cups (228 g) mixed greens

2 tablespoons (28 ml) balsamic vinegar

Heat broiler. In a food processor, puree the tomatoes, garlic, 1 tablespoon (15 ml) of the oil, and ¼ teaspoon black pepper. In 2 batches, arrange the eggplant slices on a broiler pan or baking sheet, brush with 2 tablespoons (28 ml) of the oil, and season with ¼ teaspoon black pepper. Broil until charred and tender, 3 to 4 minutes per side. Meanwhile, in a small bowl, combine the ricotta, egg substitute, basil, and ¼ teaspoon black pepper. Spread half the tomato sauce in the bottom of an 8-inch (20 cm) square baking dish. On top of it, layer a third of the eggplant slices and half the ricotta mixture. Repeat with another layer of eggplant and ricotta. Top with the remaining eggplant and tomato sauce. Sprinkle with the cheese. Reduce oven to 400°F (200°C, or gas mark 6). Bake the lasagna until bubbling, 15 to 20 minutes. Let rest for 10 minutes before serving. Divide the greens among plates and drizzle with the remaining tablespoon (15 ml) of oil, vinegar, and ¼ teaspoon of black pepper. Serve with the lasagna.

—
4 servings

Each with: 357 Calories (51% from Fat, 17% from Protein, 32% from Carb); 16 g Protein; 22 g Total Fat; 6 g Unsaturated Fat; 12 g Monounsaturated Fat; 2 g Polyunsaturated Fat; 30 g Carb; 15 g Fiber; 10 g Sugar; 311 mg Phosphorus; 382 mg Calcium; 219 mg Sodium; 1288 mg Potassium; 1338 IU Vitamin A; 72 mg ATE Vitamin E; 27 mg Vitamin C; 25 mg Cholesterol

Top of the List Vegetarian Fried Rice

When you have fried rice that tastes this good, you won't even miss the meat. Eggs add protein, and a whole lot of vegetables contribute to the nutrient levels. And the taste is superb.

¼ cup (60 ml) olive oil

1 teaspoon garlic, minced or mashed

¼ cup (25 g) green onion, diagonally sliced

¾ cup (120 g) onion, sliced

1 cup (70 g) bok choy, coarsely shredded

4 ounces (115 g) mushrooms, julienned

1 cup (145 g) snow pea pods

½ cup (120 ml) egg substitute

3 cups (585 g) brown rice, cooked and cooled

3 tablespoons (45 ml) low sodium soy sauce, or to taste

Heat wok. Add 1 tablespoon oil (15 ml) and heat. Add garlic, green onion, and regular onion and stir-fry until onions are tender. Add bok choy, mushrooms, and snow peas. Sauté 2 minutes. Remove vegetables. Add 1 tablespoon oil (15 ml) and heat. Add egg substitute. Stir until set. Remove eggs and break into very small pieces. Add remaining 2 tablespoons (28 ml) oil and add rice. Cook, stirring, until heated through. Season with soy sauce. Add vegetables and eggs and toss to mix well.

—

4 servings

Each with: 356 Calories (40% from Fat, 11% from Protein, 49% from Carb); 10 g Protein; 16 g Total Fat; 2 g Unsaturated Fat; 11 g Monounsaturated Fat; 2 g Polyunsaturated Fat; 44 g Carb; 5 g Fiber; 3 g Sugar; 217 mg Phosphorus; 65 mg Calcium; 524 mg Sodium; 465 mg Potassium; 454 IU Vitamin A; 0 mg ATE Vitamin E; 20 mg Vitamin C; 0 mg Cholesterol

On The Road to Marrakesh Stew

This spicy Moroccan stew of vegetables and dried fruit is sure to be a hit. It contains an amazing amount of flavor and great nutrition.

1 tablespoon (15 ml) olive oil

1½ cups (240 g) onion, chopped

2 garlic cloves, minced

1 teaspoon cinnamon, ground

½ teaspoon ginger, ground

½ teaspoon turmeric, ground

¼ teaspoon nutmeg, ground

¼ teaspoon red pepper, ground

2 cups (475 ml) water

3 cloves, whole

2 cups (244 g) carrot, sliced

2 cups (280 g) butternut squash, cubed

2 cups (480 g) chickpeas, cooked or canned, drained

1½ cups (200 g) sweet potatoes, cubed

½ cup (75 g) raisins

⅓ cup (43 g) dried apricots, diced

3 tablespoons (3 g) brown sugar substitute, such as Splenda

In a 4-quart (3.8 L) saucepan, heat the oil over medium-high heat. Add the onion and garlic and cook, stirring, until softened. Add the cinnamon, ginger, turmeric, nutmeg, and red pepper, stirring until absorbed. Add the water and cloves; bring to a boil. Add the carrot, squash, chickpeas, sweet potato, raisins, apricots, and brown sugar substitute and return to a boil. Reduce the heat and simmer uncovered, stirring occasionally, 40 to 45 minutes or until the sweet potato is tender.

—
4 servings

Each with: 416 Calories (13% from Fat, 11% from Protein, 77% from Carb); 12 g Protein; 6 g Total Fat; 1 g Saturated Fat; 3 g Monounsaturated Fat; 2 g Polyunsaturated Fat; 84 g Carb; 15 g Fiber; 32 g Sugar; 266 mg Phosphorus; 164 mg Calcium; 94 mg Sodium; 1261 mg Potassium; 34 916 IU Vitamin A; 0 mg ATE Vitamin E; 41 mg Vitamin C; 0 mg Cholesterol

About the Author

After being diagnosed with congestive heart failure, Dick Logue threw himself into the process of creating healthy versions of his favorite recipes. A cook since the age of twelve, he grows his own vegetables, bakes his own bread, and cans a variety of foods. He is the author of *500 Low Sodium Recipes*, *500 Low-Cholesterol Recipes*, *500 High-Fiber Recipes*, *500 Low-Glycemic-Index Recipes*, and *500 Heart-Healthy Slow Cooker Recipes*. He lives in southern Maryland.

Index